P F

MW01526925

Creating Postpartum Wellness

"No mother has to suffer from PPD needlessly. This is a fact. But until you know what you're up against, you'll still be trapped—without knowing why! A typical example is the common misconception that depression is 'all just in the mind.' (See Chapter 4: Mind-Body Connection and PPD.) Your first step is to keep an open mind; and allow Laura to take you by the hand and guide you step by step through the PPD universe. Using a 'wellness' approach, and with her usual friendly and informative style, trust me, she can help you help yourself getting out of the rut—naturally—in no time."

- Naturopath Alex Leong, B.A.S.M.

"A practical, compassionate book filled with easy-to-follow natural solutions to improve the lives of women."
- H.C. "Joe" Raymond, Certified Counselor and Life Skills Trainer
Author of *Embracing Change From The Inside Out*

"Laura Rude realizes the interconnections between mind, body, and spirit and offers down-to-earth, practical guidelines in harmonizing them."
- Karen Szillat, Early Childhood Educator and Peace Advocate
Author of *Empowering The Children: 12 Universal Values Your Child Must Learn to Succeed In Life*

"Creating Postpartum Wellness is exactly the guide you want to move from postpartum depression to postpartum happiness and good health. This book is invaluable for anyone with postpartum depression who would like an alternative treatment to prescription drugs (and a real eye-opener for anyone who thinks pharmaceuticals are the only choice.) The all-natural, simple solutions in this book are easy for any mom to implement on her own and can allow her to emerge from a dark state of depression to experience the joys of motherhood. I would encourage any new mom to read it!"

\- Theresa Callahan, Author of *Managing For Performance: Building Accountability For Team Success*

Creating Postpartum Wellness

Natural Solutions to Banish Depression after Childbirth

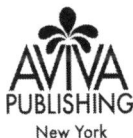

AVIVA
PUBLISHING
New York

LAURA RUDE, CHT

Creating Postpartum Wellness

Address all inquiries to:
Laura Rude
www.Postpartum-Living.com

Published by:
Aviva Publishing
Lake Placid, NY
518-523-1320
www.avivapubs.com

ISBN: 978-1-938686-36-8
Library of Congress Number: 2012924172

Editor: Michelle K. Leutzinger
Interior Layout: Liliana Gonzalez - ipublicidades.com
Cover Design: ImageTrance

Acknowledgments

First, I would like to acknowledge and thank my incredible husband, Larry. Your love and support is unwavering and your belief in me is a constant inspiration. I could not have a better husband and I feel blessed to have your enduring love and encouragement.

I am indebted to all of the mothers who have had the courage to share their experiences dealing with postpartum depression. Your bravery helps those suffering in silence to know they are not alone and understand they can get the help they need.

I want to express my appreciation to Patrick Snow, my publishing coach, who held my hand throughout the process of this book.

A good editor is vital to a good book. I am thankful to my editor, Michelle Leutzinger. Her dedication and very capable editing of the manuscript brought this book to fruition.

I would like to express my gratitude to my uplifting and encouraging friend, Theresa Callahan. Thank you for the friendship and moral support you generously provided when I needed it the most.

To all of the friends, family and colleagues who offered me love and support and believed in this book, I give you my sincere thanks.

And finally, to my amazing son, who has given me the most fulfilling job in the world—to be his mother.

Disclaimer

The information provided in this book is designed to provide helpful information on the subjects discussed. This book is not meant to be used, nor should it be used, to diagnose or treat any medical condition. For diagnosis or treatment of any medical problem, consult your physician. Any and all information contained herein is not intended to take the place of medical advice from a health care professional. Any action taken based on these contents is at the sole discretion and sole liability of the reader.

Readers should always consult appropriate health professionals on any matter relating to their health and wellbeing before taking any action of any kind concerning health-related issues. Any information or opinions provided in this book are believed to be accurate and sound; however, the author and publisher assume no liability for the use or misuse of information provided in this book, or for errors or omissions in the information contained herein. The author and publisher are not liable for any damages or negative consequences from any treatment, action, application or preparation, to any person reading or following the information in this book. References are provided for informational purposes only and do not constitute endorsement of any websites or other sources. Readers should be aware that the websites listed in this book may change.

Contents

by Diane Dean, RN

As a registered nurse, licensed professional counselor and professionally-trained coach with more than 25 years of experience, I've been witness to the growing holes in conventional healthcare, and the grave deficits in the recognition and sound treatment of women's mental health. This is especially true when worrisome symptoms arrive on the heels of a reproductive event, such as a miscarriage, abortion or a live birth. On my journey these past two decades, I've come to know two things: not everyone will seek professional treatment for their problems, and, thankfully, there are many paths to healing. These realizations led me to explore scores of non-conventional treatment techniques, such as acupuncture, massage, nutrition, energy work and naturopathy. This searching resulted in me eventually, in addition to my conventional training, becoming certified in therapeutic touch, Reiki and archetypal readings. I've had the pleasure of working alongside some of the best in the field of natural healing, namely well-renowned, internationally-known author and energy medicine expert Caroline Myss, and Shamanic expert and author Lewis Mehl-Madrona, MD. During my years working as a counselor treating women with depression and other psychological issues, tears have filled the eyes of many staring back at me, their minds full of fraught and confusion, many following the birth of their child.

In writing *Creating Postpartum Wellness,* Laura has fractured the perception that postpartum depression is a personal liability.   In her well-scripted copy, Laura:

- Works to reduce the stigma of postpartum depression

- Offers validation of the reader's struggles and experiences

- Offers hope for change

- Communicates the benefit of many varied, natural healing techniques, such as yoga, acupuncture, herbs, nutrition, hypnosis, sleep, exercise and journaling

- Offers concrete tools and strategies for recovery

Laura also weaves in crucial information about postpartum depression to educate you. If you want to take matters into your own hands, or if you want to take an active role in guiding your prescribed professional treatment, you must read *Creating Postpartum Wellness.* By offering a menu of healing choices, Laura encourages you to explore various techniques, and then she helps you determine what strategies fit best for you, your beliefs and your situation.

Had this book been available to me when I was working in a women's intensive outpatient mental health program, I would have recommended it to any women in her postpartum weeks. The recommended strategies—acupuncture, massage, yoga, aromatherapy, hypnosis, good nutrition, sleep and exercise—can not only remedy challenging times if they exist, but they just might prevent a psychological down-turn.

Through her flawless prose and supportive tone, Laura demonstrates knowledge on the subject, and she emanates enthusiasm for teaching you and helping you grow. With great courage, Laura has raised her hand when many would not. Now, maybe it's time for you to raise yours!

Diane Dean, RN-BC, LPC, CEG, is a registered nurse, a licensed counselor and a professionally trained coach with over two decades of experience in healthcare and business. Diane has taught at many colleges and universities, including the University of Pittsburgh, and she currently owns and operates Epiphany! Counseling and Wellness Center in the suburbs of Pittsburgh, PA.

Why I Wrote the Book for You

Understanding people's difficulties and—just as crucial—helping people understand their own difficulties and teaching them concrete ways to help themselves will help them better deal with their own lives, and in turn, ours.

~ KATHRYN ERSKINE, MOCKINGBIRD

I have always been interested in the different aspects of health and well-being and in how the physical and emotional aspects of a person intertwine. We human beings are both physical and emotional; one is not independent of the other. The importance of the mind-body connection became even more apparent to me once I began working with clients in my hypnotherapy practice.

I have worked with countless clients (many of whom were referred to me by medical doctors) with physical symptoms that have been largely or completely eliminated through hypnosis. In addition to utilizing hypnosis, I have helped my clients implement many of the healthy, natural methods I describe in this book that have made an enormous difference in not only their physical health but in their emotional health as well.

Having struggled with depression myself, I know the hopeless, debilitating feelings it brings, along with the tremendous guilt when you have "everything in life to be thankful for." As if the symptoms of depression aren't bad enough, adding on the guilt and shame of not bonding with this beautiful new baby, whom friends, family and society expect you to immediately bond with and feel like you're walking on clouds, can increase feelings of anguish. It can make any new mom feel like something is wrong with her. Well, something IS wrong, but it's not you—it's the postpartum depression. This depression can and will go away. If you remember nothing else during dark days, remember the word "temporary." The good news is that you are not at the mercy of your postpartum mood disorder. You do not have to sit in the misery of it, feeling helpless and hopeless. You can take charge of and get back your physical and emotional health.

Two key reasons led me to write this book of natural solutions for women with postpartum depression. First, I understood there were a variety of explanations why a woman would search for a more holistic approach to combat her PPD. Some prescription treatments for depression have adverse side effects, and some women may be concerned about what is being passed on to their baby while breast feeding. Others simply prefer to use holistic methods over pharmaceuticals. Second, I recognized that there would be fraught new mothers who would choose to do nothing rather than admit their feelings to their health care provider or therapist (or even to a spouse or friend). Many women are too ashamed or embarrassed to seek treatment. They feel they would be judged harshly if they admitted their feelings of detachment, frustration, or unhappiness toward their baby. Although there is much more awareness of PPD, and it does not carry the same stigma as it did in the past, many women still hold these fears.

For those women who want a more discreet way to treat their postpartum depression (things they can do in the privacy of their home), they can use the easy, natural, at-home methods explained in this book. For more detailed and structured help, I have created a program guide as a companion to the book, which includes a six week, step-by-step program for utilizing the natural therapies in the book. This guide includes charts and logs to make it easy for the new mother to keep track of vital information and to see her progress throughout the program. You can find more information about the guide in the back pages. One point I cannot stress enough: any woman who feels suicidal or has thoughts of hurting herself or her baby needs to seek professional help immediately. Extreme depression or violent mood swings should be addressed by a trained professional to ensure your safety and the safety of your baby.

Whatever your reason for reading this book, I'm delighted that you are taking control of your health, and I'm glad to share with you that you do have choices. There is no hard and fast rule about the best method for treating your postpartum depression. You can still implement most of the healing strategies in this book even if you also choose to take prescription medication. It is my hope that this book will be useful to all new moms, as well as their families, who seek information and a better understanding of the natural choices available to conquer postpartum depression.

Wishing you all the very best!

Laura

Who Should Read This Book

Within each of us, nature has provided all the pieces necessary to achieve exceptional health and wellness, then left it up to us to put them all together.

~ DIANE MCLAREN

If you are pregnant and looking forward to the birth of your baby, congratulations. If you have recently given birth to your baby, you are already plunging into the whirlwind of being a new mother (even if it's not your first). And if you are a relative or close friend of a new mother, you are likewise experiencing the joy and challenges of this new addition to the world.

Pregnancy is a special time for women. In most families and most situations, the birth is anticipated with delight. This is an intense and extraordinary time, as are the first months after the baby is born. You and your loved ones deserve this time to bond with the new family member and share the excitement of those first days. This is a time for mother and child to bond, for new routines and realities to form. But for too many women, postpartum depression (PPD) changes everything. If you have the baby blues or postpartum depression (including postpartum anxiety), this book is for you.

Postpartum depression falls in the middle of the spectrum of three related disorders: baby blues, postpartum depression (also known as postnatal depression) and postpartum psychosis.

The experience of baby blues is common; statistically, about 80 percent of new mothers experience a period of emotional upheaval, often depression for no reason, sadness that comes out of nowhere, tearful reactions and irritability. The baby blues usually starts within days of the birth of the child, regardless of whether the birth is of the first or subsequent child, and no matter how easy or difficult the labor was. Symptoms include trouble falling asleep or staying asleep, lack of interest in food, tension and anxiety, and possibly mood swings. Symptoms are usually mild, manageable and not so intrusive as to interfere with the enjoyment of life and the new baby. Baby blues generally only lasts approximately three weeks.

When the baby blues lasts longer than two to three weeks, or begin more than a month after the birth of the child, it is possible that the condition is developing into postpartum depression. PPD is not much different from the blues, but it is much more intense, lasts longer and can have a lasting impact on mother and baby, and on all the relationships in the mother's life. Postpartum depression can range from mild symptoms to symptoms so severe that a mother not only cannot bond with her child, she may even have disturbing thoughts and fears of harming herself or her child.

PPD does not have a single, well-understood cause. The stress of pregnancy and birth, the emotional upheaval of a new child, the physical aspects of delivery and the responsibility of caring for the infant after birth may all contribute. Other factors may include fluctuations in hormones caused by pregnancy and birth, and physical and emotional changes in the mother's life. Though the figures vary depending on the study, it is widely estimated that some 10 to 20 percent of women experience postpartum depression.

Postpartum depression typically does not arrive full-blown without warning. There are notable signs that a mother may be developing PPD or be at risk of developing the disorder. Women who have experienced a period of depression in the past may have an increased risk of developing postpartum depression, as do women who experience depression during the pregnancy.

Postpartum depression can cause sadness that seems to have no source, often accompanied by guilt because the mother expects that she should feel joyful during this special time. She can also experience emotional changes, uncontrollable negative thoughts, obsessive-compulsive behavior and physical aches and pains, as depression often manifests in the physical.

The last of the three related postnatal disorders is relatively rare and very serious. Postpartum psychosis occurs approximately once for every 500 births, more often following the birth of a first child. The disorder, thought to be a form of postpartum depression, actually resembles manic-depression or bipolar disorder. Stressors such as marital or relationship problems during pregnancy and financial concerns may contribute to this disorder, and mothers with a family history of bipolar disorder or postpartum depression may be at greater risk.

Symptoms of postpartum psychosis vary, but those that seem most common include heightened anxiety, delirium, hallucinations, euphoria, extreme mood swings, manic behavior coupled with reduced sleep, confusion, and garbled, erratic speech or the inability to speak clearly and communicate. Because of the potential for the mother to harm herself, her child or someone close to her, it is imperative to seek professional help as soon as possible. Treatment for this disorder typically requires medication and psychotherapy. While the reader should be mindful of the seriousness of this condition, prevention and treatment of postpartum psychosis is beyond the scope of this book. If you are experiencing symptoms of postpartum psychosis, do not attempt to recover alone or by the methods in this book—please seek immediate professional help.

This book is intended for you if you are a mother facing the baby blues or postpartum depression and would like to learn about and apply the wealth of natural, easy solutions that are readily available. In these pages, you will be shown a variety of methods you can implement in your recovery from postpartum depression and in the start of the next chapter of your life.

In addition to the natural methods for healing discussed in this book, I have included a few stories from women who have suffered from postpartum depression, as well as quotes from a variety of celebrity moms who have suffered and know what it's like to go through what you are going through. Any struggle can feel worse when a person believes they are different, and that no one would understand the feelings and thoughts they are experiencing. It is important for you to recognize that this happens to many new moms, and there is hope and there are solutions. Understand that you have a choice. You have many choices, actually. My hope for you as you read this book is to recognize that:

- You are not crazy and need not feel alone

- Having postpartum depression does not make you a bad mom

- You do not have to suffer in silence

- There are a variety of methods for recovery

- You have choices and options

- You will recover

Please know above all that you are not at fault and you are not alone. You can and will get through this, and I am honored to be your guide through the pages of this book to offer encouragement along the way and help you through your journey of freedom from postpartum depression.

CHAPTER 1

Sharing Their Stories

The most basic of all human needs is the need to understand and be understood. The best way to understand people is to listen to them.

~ RALPH NICHOLS

I n this first chapter, I would like to begin by introducing you to three women who suffered from postpartum depression. I am including the stories they chose to share with me as reassurance to you that perhaps the feelings you are experiencing and the thoughts that are going through your head have been experienced time and time again, not only by these three moms, but by a multitude of women before you. May their stories offer you strength and endurance as you fight, heal and recover from this mood disorder.

Sharon's Story

~

When Sharon brought her daughter home for the first time, the sun was shining and the birds were chirping. All was right with the world. She wore a smile that stretched from ear to ear and was completely content to gaze into her baby's eyes, day and sleepless night.

Sharon thought it would be the same when she brought her son home for the first time. Except that it wasn't.

Not even close.

Sharon was so excited to have her second baby. She was so excited to bring him home. But within hours of arriving safely to her house, she knew that something was wrong. She felt angry, even though she couldn't really pinpoint the source of her anger, and even though she felt she had nothing to be angry about.

What was wrong? What was going on here, Sharon wondered. Where was the bliss? Where were the chirping birds? Where were all those awesome breastfeeding hormones that had her floating on clouds?

What was so different this time, she wondered. Sharon had an eighteen-month-old to chase around this time. And her little firecracker didn't understand why she no longer had mom's undivided attention. And though it seems completely irrational now, at the time, Sharon was overwhelmed with guilt at the thought of neglecting her eighteen-month-old. She actually worried that her first-born child would stop loving her because of all the energy she was giving to the baby.

At Sharon's baby's first check-up at the pediatrician's office, they noticed some warning signs, and gave her a multiple-choice questionnaire to confirm she was suffering from Postpartum Depression. Sharon thought, "No, that couldn't happen to me." She was sure that she would pass with flying colors. Yes, she had her issues, but depression? She would not admit that. No way.

Sharon's test revealed she had postpartum depression. In fact, it was so severe that the doctor and nurses buzzed around "like I was an eggshell strapped with explosives," she said. She wanted to go home. She begged to go home. And they wouldn't let her. She was beginning to feel like a white van and a straightjacket might be waiting in the parking lot. Sharon was fed lunch and then asked to wait while they found a doctor (one who wasn't a pediatrician) for her to talk to.

Finally she did talk to the other doctor. The doctor confirmed that Sharon was suffering from postpartum depression and exhaustion and expressed to Sharon what a dangerous combination that could be. The doctor then asked Sharon's husband to join them and gently scolded him for letting her do too much. The doctor explained, in complicated medical terms, that Sharon needed to get some sleep.

The next few months were rough for Sharon. She tried to prioritize resting. She tried to come to terms with the fact that not everything was peachy the second time around.

After months of dealing with anger, anxiety, exhaustion and depression, Sharon eventually did begin to feel better, but she remembers wondering during that time if she would ever be herself again.

Susan's Story

~

Susan had difficulty getting pregnant for years. When she found out she was going to have a baby, she was elated and eagerly anticipated the baby's arrival.

Susan went into labor surrounded by loved ones at the hospital and gave birth to her healthy, precious baby.

Soon after leaving the hospital, Susan's elation turned to sadness. She couldn't understand what was wrong. She knew she should be happy. This baby was a true blessing and it made no sense to be sad.

Susan kept everything locked inside, too ashamed to share her feelings with anyone.

As the weeks passed, Susan began to feel even worse. It was difficult to get out of bed. She cried for what seemed like no reason and found herself repeatedly getting angry with her husband.

What should have been one of the best times of her life became a time filled with guilt for not being happy. As the guilt grew, she became more sullen.

She felt so alone. The more alone she felt, the more she withdrew from those around her. Holding the baby just made her cry.

Six weeks after giving birth, Susan's husband drove her and the baby to the doctor's office for the baby's six week check-up. As they were speeding down the highway, the thought came over her to unbuckle her seat belt, open the door, and jump out. Surely at these high speeds she would hit her head after she fell from the car and it would all be over.

She turned this idea over in her mind for several minutes, replaying the scene again and again. It took an unbelievable amount of courage to talk herself out of doing it.

Susan looked over at her husband and then to her beautiful baby in the back seat, and finally realized she needed help.

Camilla's Story

~

Since puberty, Camilla had suffered from bouts of depression and anxiety. At twenty-two, she was diagnosed with dysthymic disorder, and at twenty-five, she was diagnosed with premenstrual depressive disorder (PMDD). Depression, anxiety, and OCD ran in her family for all of the generations she knew, and she was no stranger to the effects of mental illness. However, she had been able to control her depression and anxiety with exercise, meditation, relaxation, and proper diet until she gave birth to her first child.

Camilla conceived naturally at the age of twenty-seven. She and her husband were both incredibly happy about the news, and her pregnancy passed mostly uneventfully. She did experience a bout of mild antenatal depression in her first trimester, but this passed as she entered her second trimester. During her pregnancy, she took an organic prenatal vitamin and a prenatal DHA supplement as a means for preventing PPD. She had a natural birth in a reputable private hospital, and she went home with her son in twenty-four hours.

In the first two weeks after her son arrived, Camilla began to experience the effects of postpartum depression, OCD, and anxiety. She had a depressed mood, a feeling of detachment from her child, and unavoidable, graphic, intrusive fears about harm coming to her child. When she asked her doula and her OB about what she was experiencing, she was told it was the "typical baby blues." Her anxiety increased, and her intrusive thoughts overtook most of the days of her maternity leave from work.

Camilla suffered silently and brushed her worrying emotions aside. Finally, when her child was four months old, Camilla realized that she was, in fact, suffering from full-blown postpartum depression, and decided to take action.

Celebrity Moms Who Have Struggled

Many celebrity moms have struggled with a postpartum mood disorder. As you read the experiences of these famous mothers, my desire is for you to gain a feeling of hope and optimism. These women have gone through the nasty experience of postpartum depression in front of an audience, and have come out the other side. An overwhelming number of other women whom you don't know have also struggled. You may also be astonished by the number of moms you actually *do* know who have wrestled with PPD, but have chosen to keep their experiences to themselves.

"I felt like a zombie. I couldn't access my heart. I couldn't access my emotions. I couldn't connect. It was terrible."

Gwyneth Paltrow

"I think if there is any goal in me talking about it, it would be to eradicate the shame around it. It's just what happens sometimes and, for me, I just waited way too long to reach out for help."

Alanis Morissette

"My abilities to cope, problem solve, and adjust to new situations, abilities that had served me so well, were beyond my reach."

Valerie Plame Wilson

"[My husband] would ask what he could do to help, but knowing there was nothing he could do, I screamed expletives at him, behavior he had never experienced in the seven years we had been together."

Bryce Dallas Howard

"I cried all day over everything."

Carnie Wilson

"PPD is out of their control, but the treatment and healing process is not."

Brooke Shields

"I had just given birth to this perfect baby, but absolutely nothing made me happy anymore. I had no idea what was wrong. I had these great blessings, but I felt empty. I'd put Ava in her crib and go outside and scream for a minute."

Melissa Rycroft

"[It] all came crashing down the second [Frankie] was born. I want to be honest about it because I think there's still so much shame when you have mixed feelings about being a mom instead of feeling this sort of 'bliss.'"

Amanda Peet

CHAPTER 2

What Is Postpartum Depression?

Time and health are two precious assets that we don't recognize and appreciate until they have been depleted.

~ DENIS WAITLEY

When defining postpartum depression (PPD), perhaps the most important part of the definition is the word temporary. You should think of PPD as a temporary setback along the way to a happy future with your new baby and your family.

Technically, postpartum depression is an actual medical diagnosis. It is a disorder and it can happen to any new mother, whether she's having her first child or her fourth.

By definition, postpartum depression is a moderate to severe form of depression that can affect a new mother, starting any time after the birth of her child. It can last a few weeks, a few months, or it can last for a year or longer. Where the baby blues can last two or three weeks, bringing with it an emotional rollercoaster, unexpected and unexplained mood swings and sadness, when the blues continue past three weeks, it's possible the mother is developing postpartum depression...

If you think you may be seeing signs of postpartum depression in yourself or in your partner, remember that it's a temporary condition—and that you're not alone.

Every woman is different, but there are times when it is possible to at least prepare for the possibility of PPD, because genetic history and personal history or current living situations indicate the mother may experience the disorder. The CDC indicates that young mothers under the age of 20 may be more likely to develop PPD, as are single mothers, women who are under a great deal of stress, those experiencing financial stress or stresses within their relationships, women whose pregnancy was unplanned and women who have suffered from depression in the past.

Recognizing Postpartum Depression Symptoms

Postpartum depression is essentially a more intense, longer-lasting version of the baby blues. Its symptoms do not differ considerably from any other depressive experience. Notable symptoms include:

- Lethargy, difficulty in performing routine tasks, lack of interest in keeping up appearance

- Fatigue, exhaustion

- Insomnia or hypersomnia (sleeping too much)

- An inability to bond or care for the new baby

- Mood swings

- Unexplained sadness or crying

- Anxiety, nervousness, tension

- Feelings of guilt or worthlessness, feeling like all the pleasures in life are gone

- Pain

Symptoms of PPD vary between women, but emotional changes are constant with the disorder. Erratic emotions can vary from extreme joy to despondency within minutes, leaving a new mother confused and often feeling ashamed or guilty—this is supposed to be a wonderful time in her life and the lives of her family members, but she's dealing with inexplicable mood swings.

As with any form of depression, the mood swings and sadness of PPD can make it hard for a new mother to even want to carry out all the tasks that come with everyday life, let alone take on the responsibilities of having a new child. Depression brings with it fatigue and lethargy, so even if she's not sleep deprived, the new mother may not feel like taking care of herself and taking care of her child may feel like a monumental chore. Fatigue and lethargy can stand in the way of a mother bonding with her new infant, and can make her resent the care she has to take with the child, which can throw another barrier up between mother and child.

For many women, irritability is part and parcel of PPD, causing rifts between partners and possibly causing friends and family to withdraw from her at a time when she could really use everyone in her support system to stay close.

The emotional rollercoaster of postpartum depression can mimic a diagnosis of Bipolar Disorder and in fact, women whose family medical history includes relatives with bipolar disorder may be predisposed to PPD.

Postpartum depression can also bring with it a form of Obsessive-Compulsive Disorder (OCD), which can manifest as repetitive behaviors or recurring thoughts. Many mothers with PPD-induced OCD find themselves obsessively cleaning their surroundings and guarding their baby from harm to a paranoid extent. The mother may experience reoccurring fear that something is going to hurt her child, or that something she has done—or hasn't done—will cause danger to her child.

Even more frightening among the repetitive thoughts is the fear that the mother will harm herself or her new child. Some women find themselves thinking about suicide, even if they've never had any desire to die. According to the CDC there are some 950,000 cases of PPD in the U.S. every year. Of those, mothers who actually follow through on obsessive thoughts of hurting themselves or their children are extremely rare. However, this is a symptom a mother needs to address with her doctor without delay.

Not all the symptoms of postpartum depression are emotional or mental. As a television commercial informs, "Depression hurts." PPD can bring with it aches and pains; backaches, headaches, stomach aches and joint pain are not uncommon for people experiencing depression. The anxiety and tension associated with PPD can cause chest pain, sometimes leading the mother to believe she's having a heart attack. As with any depression, the headache is not a tumor; the chest pain is not a heart attack. They are physical manifestations of psychological disturbances.

Postpartum Depression, Family and Friends

While it may be a special time in a woman's life, having a new baby in the home is stressful. Routines change or disintegrate altogether, noise and confusion is commonplace, sleep schedules are disrupted and financial concerns are frequent. A new mother struggling with PPD has even bigger challenges as she fights depression, lethargy and a rollercoaster of emotions.

This is a time when a good, solid relationship is crucial. However, it is also a time that can put a lot of stress on a marriage or partnership. From the family's perspective, living with someone who is experiencing depression is a challenge no matter what the other circumstances are. From inside the depression, it is difficult for the woman to acknowledge the love she may feel for the people around her. It is hard to be appreciative of what her husband and family and friends are doing to help out, and just as hard to accept that help. With the feelings of guilt and worthlessness that accompany the PPD, the woman may think that if she were any good whatsoever, she'd be handling all the responsibilities herself. Surely she can handle an infant who weighs less than 10 pounds on top of all her usual responsibilities—she's Wonder Woman, right?

Managing expectations is important in managing the disorder—and it's not just the mother's expectations of herself that need tempering. Husbands, partners, family members and friends in her life may not understand that the changes postpartum depression has brought about are not forever. What the husband sees is a wife who is unhappy or downright miserable, unsociable and uncaring and sometimes unkempt. She's not interested in all the things she used to care about, and doesn't seem to take pleasure in anything or anyone. There's a good chance she's not taking care of herself, and a chance she's not taking care of their child. It's hard for a husband or partner to understand and harder still to realize it's only temporary.

Postpartum Depression and YOU

If you're suffering from postpartum depression, it might feel like all the light and love have disappeared from your life. Every day is an effort to get through, and previously pleasurable pursuits like reading, watching movies, working out, shopping, spending time with family, or talking to friends can all seem empty and meaningless.

Postpartum depression robs you of the energy you need to beat back fatigue and meet goals, to accomplish chores and enjoy life. Because you're not performing up to pre-baby levels, you may start feeling worthless. If depression has stolen your libido, you may feel unattractive, even if you're the one turning down amorous adventures with your partner.

Depression isn't reasonable—it doesn't allow you to look at the spiral that started with fatigue, lead to not wanting sex, continued to not dressing up and grooming, and led you to feel unattractive and worthless for not having a relationship with your partner. Depression just puts up big signs that read NO and STOP and GIVE UP.

Because you are at the center of the PPD, you will be the one experiencing most deeply the negative thoughts and unrealistic expectations (because really, adding a new child into the existing routine is going to change things and is going to add work and is going to make everything harder). You may feel relationships with friends and family members slipping and worry that there are going to be long-term consequences. It may take some time for the effects of PPD to lift, but as you will discover in this book, there are healing options available, and there are things you can do to take back control of your own life and emotions. There are natural and easy solutions that can help you combat the effects of postpartum depression.

Postpartum depression doesn't have to keep you from enjoying the beginning of your life with your new child.

Understanding Postpartum Depression

The causes of postpartum depression are not completely understood by medical science, but there are a number of factors that seem to be involved. Pregnancy causes significant physical changes to a woman's body, and labor activates and depletes many hormones. Emotional changes can be the result of stressors, hormones, or even your situation at the time of birth.

Some of the emotional causes behind PPD can be from feeling uncomfortable and self-conscious in your new body. Pregnancy weight and the changes pregnancy can cause might make you feel unattractive. If it's been difficult to be intimate with your partner during the pregnancy or following a difficult birth, that lack of intimacy can also make you feel less attractive and less confident.

For a new mother, concerns about her ability to fulfill her role as a mom can have a heavy impact on self-esteem. Just taking care of a new baby can cause anxiety and stress, from the demands on time and energy to the fear of doing it wrong and harming the child.

Physically, a difficult birth can lead to depression, as can the pain after the birth.

Physical Changes to Your Body

After a woman gives birth, levels of estrogen, progesterone and cortisol can fluctuate dramatically, which can have an effect on mood and energy levels. The fluctuation of hormones in the body can make it difficult to lose the pregnancy weight and the changes in body appearance can lead to depression.

Depression also has an effect on hormone levels. Depression can lead to an increase in levels of the hormone cortisol, a stress hormone which can act to suppress the immune system at a time when you could really use all your body's defense systems to be working for you. Although medical science doesn't understand exactly why, there are often elevated levels of cortisol in the blood after a birth.

Additionally, women lose nutrients during pregnancy and delivery. Studies show that nutritional deficiencies including iron, zinc, the B vitamins, selenium and calcium, and omega-3 fatty acids can contribute to postpartum depression.

Insufficient and Interrupted Sleep

Another culprit in the development of PPD is thought to be the change in the mother's sleep patterns following the birth of a baby. Sleep deprivation can lead to depression. For a mother of a newborn who is just hoping to catch four straight hours of sleep followed by some significant naps, sleep is at a premium. Making matters worse, depression can bring with it disturbances to the sleep cycle, causing interrupted sleep, insomnia or hypersomnia.

Stress

In addition to psychological and physiological impacts, a stressful home life or environment can increase the likelihood of PPD, as can a lack of social support.

A stressful marriage can become further stressed with the arrival of a new baby. If you're already missing the closeness or experiencing tension in your relationship, the additional stresses of pregnancy and birth and the new little person may be enough to bring on postpartum depression.

Financial stresses can also contribute to the likelihood of a mother developing PPD. Worrying about where the money will come from to take care of a child who is totally dependent on you along with existing financial concerns adds another layer of stress at a busy time during your life.

Not all the stresses associated with a new baby are negative. The stress of adding a child to an existing household is usually positive, but it's still a stress. Any changes at this point in your life can be stressful—leaving a job to become a mother, or taking a leave and suddenly not having a job, can be disconcerting

Moving Forward

When you're in the grip of depression, one of the hardest things to do is to take a step forward. One of the coping techniques taught by behavioral psychotherapy is opposite action. What this means is, when the depression urges you to curl up into a ball and watch television, ignoring the tasks and responsibilities hanging over you (and consequently making you feel worse after your temporary hiatus away from the To Do list), instead you must get up and do one thing. Just one. Sometimes it's the most difficult thing you have to tackle that day. Sometimes it's the easiest—but procrastination, depression and lethargy have made it feel enormous.

Opposite action also means taking action. Instead of sitting, stand. Instead of watching television, listen to upbeat music. Instead of watching the world go by without you in it, go for a walk—your baby will benefit from the closeness of the two of you out in the world and the natural sunlight is good for everybody's mood.

Throughout the rest of this book you'll have a chance to find strategies and solutions that work for you as you move through your postpartum depression and into a happier future with your family.

CHAPTER 3

Overcoming the Stigma of Postpartum Depression— Managing Expectations and Taking Action

You gain strength, courage, and confidence by every experience in which you really stop to look fear in the face. You must do the thing which you think you cannot do.

~ ELEANOR ROOSEVELT

One of the contributing factors to postpartum depression is often a feeling of guilt. New mothers generally anticipate the birth of a baby and our society builds the anticipation with gifts and showers from friends, happy advertisements in every form of media, and cards, letters, emails and phone calls from well-wishing family and friends. The message, which the new mother receives through countless avenues, is that she has every reason to be happy.

When the birth is difficult or the child is born with a health condition or the mother's health is negatively affected by the pregnancy or birth, friends and family may anticipate that the mother could become depressed or may be experiencing uncertain, erratic emotions. But when a healthy child is born to a healthy mother, friends and family who have not experienced postpartum depression for themselves may not understand what the mother is going through. Casual comments can impact a depressed mother far beyond what was meant— "cheer up," "count your blessings," "but everything is wonderful" can leave you feeling more depressed than ever.

Opposite Action

Opposite action is as simple as it sounds, and it's effective at helping to relieve some of the symptoms of depression, but it does require awareness. At its most basic, opposite action is a behavioral technique utilized by cognitive therapists to help patients suffering from depression become aware of their moods and then take actual, active steps to, essentially, defy them.

The technique requires you to be aware of what you're thinking and feeling in the moment, which may require charting your moods on paper. A simple calendar or grid allows you to track your emotions at any given time of day. Once you've learned to identify what you're feeling rather than letting your emotions have their way with you, you can make conscious decisions to change your situation.

Sometimes breaking through the depression, even temporarily, can help. Simply identifying that you feel sad and that you're putting off what you need to do and giving in to the depression can help you break out of the downward spiral. Putting off what you need to be doing can lead to more depression as well as feelings of guilt, shame or worthlessness, but in the grips of depression, sometimes taking those steps just feels too hard.

Recognizing what you're feeling can help. Once you've identified that you're feeling unhappy or lethargic, and are in the moment, aware of your actions, you change them. Bringing yourself into the moment means paying attention—if you feel scattered and distant from yourself, do something to bring yourself back. Wash your hands. Brush your teeth. Make a cup of tea and observe all the steps you take. Put on hand lotion and notice what it feels like to rub the lotion into your skin.

Then try taking a simple step to change the mood. The change you make can be as small as getting up and walking into another room, or turning on music you love, or reading a book for a few minutes. It can be going outside long enough to feel the sunshine on your face or the cool breeze on your skin. It's something that breaks up the rhythm the depression has created, and it can make the depression lift enough for you to take other steps.

Like calling a friend and asking for help. Asking for help may be as simple as asking a friend or relative to sit with the baby at nap time so you can take a nap yourself, or take a walk around the block and clear your head, or indulge in a little alone time by doing some gentle yoga stretches in another room, while your child is safe and in good hands.

You can also ask for help by letting your friends know you're ready for some companionship. You've just had a baby—you don't have to remain isolated from the rest of the world. If you're not comfortable going out yet, ask your friends and family to come visit. If you're worried about your mood because of sadness or irritability while company's still there, no one will find it strange for a new mother to cut a visit short because she's tired and needs to rest.

Expectations—Yours, and Those of Others

Compounding the emotional upheaval of postpartum depression is the fact that it's not well understood, and it's not well discussed. Many women, whether they understand they're probably experiencing postpartum depression or not, choose not to talk about it to their spouse, their family or their friends, and possibly not even to their doctor.

Unfortunately, there is still a stigma attached to postpartum depression. In part, because it is a diagnosable disorder, there's a feeling that it brings with it the label of mental illness. Women are afraid of being judged "crazy" and being considered an unfit mother. A new mom going through PPD needs all the support she can get, and she is likely hiding the symptoms and denying herself—and her family—the help she needs.

Postpartum depression is not a defect or a failing, but there may be people in your life who don't understand this mood disorder and, whether judging or trying (ineffectively) to help, offer suggestions along the line of "Snap out of it!" or "Count your blessings, look on the bright side!" Being perceived to be complaining about imagined problems may keep a woman from asking for help.

Putting on a brave front and hiding depression can backfire. If you're hoping that someone will notice that you're overwhelmed and you need help, but you're still accomplishing everything on the To Do list, taking care of your child and telling everyone there's nothing wrong, it's possible that no one will reach out to help, which will only make you feel more isolated and overwhelmed. Some women hide their PPD so well that even their husbands don't see the symptoms of depression. If a husband doesn't know his wife is melting down, it's harder for him to offer help, and harder for him to understand why she's asking (if she does). Just managing to ask for help might be the step that alerts friends and family to what you're feeling.

Hiding the symptoms of postpartum depression makes the disorder seem more rare than it actually is, and makes it that much harder to talk about.

Societal Expectations

Society as a whole seems to expect that a new mother will simply carry on with her life—the new child will simply add to the mix of her existing responsibilities and she will happily charge forth. Popular media contribute additional unrealistic expectations. The slick, shiny magazine ads with smiling mothers and babies present a sunny world of motherhood. A new mother, confronted with the 24/7 reality of a newborn who frequently cries, may think she's failing because of unreasonable, media-invented expectations. A new mother may find herself resenting the sudden, all-consuming responsibility of motherhood, and can feel like a failure rather than a real-life mom.

Don't let the stigma of being perceived as a bad mother, or as mentally ill, cause you to hide your postpartum depression. Postpartum depression is temporary, but you don't have to lose this time with your new baby. You deserve to be happy. Postpartum depression is a diagnosis, a real disorder, and you can fight it.

CHAPTER 4

Mind-Body Connection and Postpartum Depression

Health is a state of complete harmony of the body, mind and spirit. When one is free from physical disabilities and mental distractions, the gates of the soul open.

~ B. K. S. IYENGAR

Some of us live in our heads, intellectualizing everything and viewing the body as nothing more than a container and transporter for the mind. Others are far less introspective, not taking much time to consider what the mind might be doing, beyond its role in whatever physical endeavor they are pursuing.

The truth is, mind and body are connected and what affects one, affects the other. Stress, pain, fear, anxiety and negative emotions all have an effect on your body, as do joy, anticipation and contentment. Therefore, taking care of the body is just as important as taking care of the emotional aspects of PPD. That is why later in this book we will address breathing, hypnosis, journaling and a variety of other natural solutions to coping with and overcoming postpartum depression, as well as information on eating right and supplementing your diet with vitamins and minerals.

The mind-body connection describes the way that thoughts can affect your physical body and your physical condition can affect how you feel emotionally. Have you ever pleaded sickness to get out of an event (or a day at work) and then found you really don't feel well? Or have you found yourself coming down with a headache or backache because you're faced with a series of unpleasant tasks or an event you'd rather avoid?

The mind-body connection works in both directions. Your thoughts carry energy that can affect your health, and physical injury or illness can make you feel weary. The connection is one reason so many people get sick during stressful times in their lives—the body's response to stress can be headache, backache, ulcer—even the common cold. Medical science will likely never cure the common cold, partly because there are so many variations of the viruses that cause colds, but also because we cannot completely eliminate stress from our lives at all times. In a way, colds are nature's way of telling us to scale back and relax.

There are ways to use the connection between mind and body to improve your emotional and physical state when you're fighting postpartum depression. Some do so by targeting the mind, including hypnosis and subliminal recordings as well as relaxation and meditation techniques (see *Chapter 11: Hypnosis—Using the Power of Your Mind;* and *Chapter 12: Take a Break—Relaxation and Stress Management*). Other methods target the body, namely diet and exercise (see *Chapter 7: Healthy Diet—You're Still Eating for Two;* and *Chapter 10: Make Your Move—Exercise and Depression*). I recommend incorporating both approaches at once.

When you're struggling to overcome postpartum depression, you're struggling with a mood disorder that has its own diagnosis and its own, not clearly understood causes. You need every weapon in your arsenal so you can fight back and come out on top. That means putting your body to work along with your mind to combat your PPD.

Pain and Postpartum Depression

Those ads that claim "depression hurts" have actual medical evidence to back them up. Research regarding how the central nervous system and neuropathways of the body work shows that physical and mental pain use the same pathways through the body. There's no differentiation between the pain of an injury and the pain of a loss. Because of this, it should come as no surprise that the chemicals at play during depression (largely the stress hormones and neurotransmitters) can cause physical symptoms, such as:

- Back pain, neck pain, joint pain
- Changes in appetite—not eating or overeating
- Weight gain or weight loss
- Chest pain, palpitations (racing heartbeat)
- Constipation or diarrhea
- Fatigue
- Headaches and stomach aches
- High blood pressure
- Sleeping too much or too little
- Sexual problems
- Shortness of breath

People seeking treatment for depression are apt to downplay their physical symptoms, believing that everything that seems physical is actually all in their minds. They perceive seeking help for the physical symptoms as complaining, but it's not complaining— it's understanding. Rather than fighting to ignore the symptoms and putting energy into explaining (to yourself, your doctor, your friends and family) that you're only facing emotional symptoms, admitting that the physical pain exists can actually help relieve that pain. In addition, persistent physical pain can make it more difficult to get out from under the pain of postpartum depression.

Talking to your doctor about the physical symptoms of PPD can help the two of you create a treatment plan that addresses both the physical and the emotional aspects of your depression.

Talking to your doctor can help you rule out any physical problems that may exist in addition to (or exacerbating) your postpartum depression, which can help set your mind at ease. In addition, you may be able to find safe and effective ways to deal with the physical pain, which in turn will help you feel better emotionally while you fight the PPD.

Another way of putting this is: if pain can cause depression, an absence of pain can help alleviate depression. If depression can cause physical pain—and reports say that it can—working to lift the depression can help with the physical pain as well.

Neurotransmitters and Postpartum Depression

Neurotransmitters are nature's anti-depressants, so to speak. According to medical science, the top three neurotransmitters in the brain are serotonin, norepinephrine and dopamine. Neurotransmitters are neurochemicals that transmit nerve impulses, or chemical messages to the body and mind. When these three agents are out of balance, both depression and physical pain can occur.

One of the best ways to modulate your neurotransmitters is to exercise. Exercise helps flush the body of anxiety chemicals like cortisol and adrenaline and encourages the release of feel-good hormones like endorphins. Additionally, exercise causes the brain to secrete neurotransmitters, which essentially function as antidepressants. See *Chapter 10: Make Your Move—Exercise and Depression* for more detailed information on exercise and postpartum depression.

Diet and Postpartum Depression

Diet and postpartum depression go hand in hand as part of the mind-body connection. The body needs healthy fuel to function properly, both physically and emotionally. Of course, it is often difficult to eat a balanced, healthy diet while incorporating a new baby into the household, along with everything else that's coming your way.

The good news is the changes you can make to help short-circuit PPD and start eating healthy are fairly simple—reduce your consumption of junk food; increase your intake of fish, fruits and vegetables. See *Chapter 7: Healthy Diet—You're*

Still Eating for Two for more detailed information on diet and postpartum depression.

Pregnancy, Hormones and Postpartum Depression

Pregnancy changes hormone levels throughout your body. During pregnancy, estrogen and progesterone are present in larger than normal levels which drop back to normal levels within 24 hours of giving birth. Some researchers believe that the sudden drop in these hormones can trigger postpartum depression.

Levels of thyroid hormones may also drop after giving birth. Thyroid hormones regulate how the body stores and releases caloric energy from food, and low thyroid can cause depression.

Self-esteem and Postpartum Depression

The changes in your body from the pregnancy, the baby weight you might still be carrying, and the variety of new tasks you're trying to juggle can make it hard to maintain self-confidence and self-esteem. You might feel less attractive or less capable of things you used to do easily, like juggling a busy schedule.

Like other matters related to the mind-body connection, self-esteem and self-confidence can be built back up by taking physical action, whether that's finding an exercise routine, getting out of the house, or joining a new class. Hybrid education that allows online classes coupled with on-campus time might be perfect for a new mother who needs to get out sometimes and other times needs to stay in. At the same time, it allows you to learn something new and meet a few new people. Taking on new challenges such as classes can help bolster sagging confidence. Likewise, exercise can stimulate feelings of accomplishment and pride, as well as help you lose weight.

CHAPTER 5

Natural Treatment Options for Postpartum Depression

The best and most efficient pharmacy is within your own system.
~ ROBERT C. PEALE

G iving birth has changed significantly in the last half century. If you want a pop culture reference, take a look at any of the sitcoms or movies from the 1950s—Lucy Ricardo in "I Love Lucy" went off to have her baby in isolation while Ricky, who was experiencing sympathetic labor pains, certainly was not in the delivery room. Compare that to Rachel giving birth to Emma in "Friends" in the 21st century—she had her friends surrounding her until the last minute and the father of her child talking her though labor.

Giving birth is regarded as a natural experience— maybe too much so. Who hasn't heard a reference to women giving birth and going right back to a different kind of labor the same day, hunting down a saber tooth tiger or toiling away in the fields? If you've just had a baby, you know better. If you had a difficult pregnancy, then such references may well be offensive to you.

Having a baby is a significant event and your body experiences trauma. It is not surprising that this can be followed by depression, as the stress surrounding the birth and the reality that your life has changed forever hits home.

What might be surprising is how different your experience as a new mother may be from what you anticipated. This may make your struggle with PPD difficult to accept.

Don't be so hard on yourself. Give yourself a break—literally. One of the most often overlooked natural solutions to postpartum depression is giving yourself permission to let a few things slide—the housework; dinner on the table, promptly and every night; your career. There really isn't a requirement for you to add in the responsibility of a new baby while keeping everything else going exactly the way it was. Just for now, take a break and treat yourself as an individual who has just had an experience that no one else can have. Your experience of giving birth is yours alone—no one else could have had it. Your recovery from PPD is the same—no one else will experience everything the same way you do, and what works for everyone else may not be right for you. The contrary may hold true as well; solutions that others swear by may in fact be the answer to your postpartum depression symptoms.

So, please, give yourself a break and give yourself permission to take the time to get well again. You, your partner, your new baby, your entire family—you all deserve this time together and to consider the best solutions to help you overcome postpartum depression.

This book contains chapters covering healthy diet strategies, how to use hypnosis to improve your health both physically and emotionally, ways to naturally regulate your hormones, vitamins and supplements you may be lacking, the importance of exercise, relaxation and stress management techniques, light therapy, as well as chapters on journaling and the importance of sleep—and how to get some during this busy, challenging time of your life. Charts and logs are included in the Appendix to help you track your steps and measure your progress.

Why Natural?

Natural solutions are those found largely outside western medicine. Western medicine, also known as traditional, orthodox or allopathic medicine, is widely accepted today as "modern medicine". Many consider it the only path to turn to, but it is worth remembering that herbal medicine and homeopathic treatments were widely used until sometime in the 20th century. Today, some medical schools are beginning to expand their teachings to include traditions from countries that use what western medicine considers alternative, natural or homeopathic treatments.

Naturopathic medicine treats the body as a whole, integrating the mind-body connection, and regards the patient in her entirety and not simply as a collection of symptoms that need to be treated and dismissed. Naturopathic medicine accepts the idea that the body holds the key to healing within itself.

Natural solutions look at the cause of the disease or disorder as well as how to treat it. Natural medicine takes into account a person's mind and body, lifestyle and habits, diet and exercise, stressors and tension releasers.

Natural solutions for healing take into account the idea that the body has healing mechanisms of its own that can be brought to bear by making changes in lifestyle and behaviors (including eating behaviors, exercise, relaxation and the like). Naturopathic doctors also bring medical science solutions into the mix. The idea is not to turn away from modern medicine, but to find the combination of techniques and solutions that treat the patient as a whole.

Alternative medicine can fall into the natural medicine arena, using alternative therapies (either alternative to western medicine or complementary to it) such as acupuncture, hypnosis, biofeedback, chiropractic techniques, massage therapy and yoga. Herbal and homeopathic remedies can offer healing as quickly, efficiently and thoroughly in many cases as western medicine's pharmaceutical treatments. To achieve this high degree of efficacy, such remedies must be manufactured and controlled by knowledgeable manufacturers using accepted techniques. Natural remedies can be just as potent as pharmaceutical remedies, thus it is important to have the proper information on dosage and use.

The Mind-Body Connection Revisited

Among the reasons natural solutions can be effective for battling postpartum depression is that natural solutions key in to the mind-body connection. Exercise, which can be as simple as waltzing around the living room with your new baby, or as complex as finding a gym with good childcare and taking up body sculpting, will free up endorphins in your body. Those same chemicals that give you your "second wind" when you "hit the wall" in training are freed up by a good workout.

A healthier body will also help you feel better emotionally. This is a win-win situation for both mind and body.

The same mind-body connection is why diet factors in. Eating a healthy diet and eating regularly throughout the day are simple and natural ways to fuel your body, maintain even blood sugar levels, and, as most people already recognize, improve mental health.

Techniques

Relaxation and stress management techniques such as meditation, yoga, and aromatherapy can help you combat stressors that send the body into fight-or-flight mode (a biological response of animals to acute stress) and that trigger stress hormones such as cortisol and adrenaline (see *Chapter 4: The Mind-Body Connection and Postpartum Depression*). Meditation can also help you increase the levels of serotonin, norepinephrine and dopamine in your system. These are neurotransmitters that, when balanced, act as natural shields against depression.

Sleep is a natural defense against depression and Chapter 17 will discuss natural solutions for finding and attaining better sleep. Sleep and depression are related according to length of sleep and soundness of sleep, which scientists are able to measure. In another example of the mind-body relationship, physical exercise may not help a new mother find the time to get more sleep, but it can help her make the most of the sleep she gets. Physical exercise leads the body to deeper, better quality sleep.

CHAPTER 6

Informing Your Healthcare Provider

Your present circumstances don't determine where you can go; they merely determine where you start.

~ NIDO QUBEIN

It is important to keep your family doctor or ob/gyn in the loop when you are experiencing symptoms of PPD and taking natural steps to combat it. Visiting your doctor is the most logical place to start.

If your symptoms have not faded within a few weeks, as is common for the baby blues, or if your symptoms are getting worse, you need to see your doctor without delay.

When preparing for your doctor's appointment to discuss postpartum depression, you can take some steps ahead of time to ensure a productive appointment. Preparing in advance is especially important if you are experiencing confusion or memory loss as part of your PPD—that way you don't forget to tell your doctor the important details.

1. Write down what you've been feeling, and when you first started feeling that way (see the Edinburgh Postnatal Depression Scale included at the end of this chapter, which can help you summarize your emotional symptoms so that you can be clear and concise with your doctor). The scale tracks mood over one week's time for an accurate picture of symptoms.

2. If you've ever been diagnosed with another depressive episode or mental health disorder, this is not the time to be shy. Your medical records are confidential. Share your conditions with your doctor.

3. If you've previously been on an antidepressant, record when you were on the drug, which antidepressant it was, how long you were on it, whether or not you used any other types of antidepressants, and any side effects or problems you may have experienced.

4. Make a list of all over-the-counter medicines you are taking, as well as any herbal therapies. If you were taking any before your pregnancy, and stopped, include those in the list. Also list the vitamins and supplements you take.

5. Write down the questions you want to ask your doctor and the points you want to make. It's easy to forget during the appointment itself if you feel rushed, or if you're uncomfortable.

6. If you're comfortable doing so, bring a friend or relative who can help you provide information to your doctor. They can also help you to remember and make sense of what you were told after your appointment.

Some of the questions you will want to ask your doctor include: what is his or her diagnosis, whether or not he or she believes you have postpartum depression, and whether your doctor will be looking into physical causes for symptoms.

When discussing treatment options with your doctor, you may want to ask about the natural solutions you are interested in. If your appointment is with your family doctor or ob/gyn, there is no reason not to ask about natural treatments as well as what western medicine may have to offer. If you intend to make changes to your diet or exercise levels or start an herbal therapy, you will want to consult your doctor before making these changes, especially if you are breastfeeding.

The Diagnosis

The Edinburgh Postnatal Depression Scale included at the end of this chapter can help you track your symptoms and enable your doctor to better understand what it is you're experiencing.

Some of the questions your doctor is likely to ask you, and for which you may want to jot down notes before your appointment, are:

- When did your symptoms first develop and how long have you had them?

- Have your symptoms been getting worse?

- How much sleep have you been able to get and what is the quality of that sleep?

- Are you experiencing insomnia or hypersomnia (sleeping too much)?

- Have you experienced any changes in energy levels?

- Have you experienced any changes in appetite (increase or decrease)?

- Have you felt irritable, anxious, and/or have you been experiencing mood swings?

- Do you currently have significant stress in your relationship, finances, or in another area of your life?

- Have you previously been diagnosed with any medical conditions, either physical or mental?

- Have you ever been in therapy and if so, did you feel it was useful?

If your doctor recommends antidepressants as a treatment plan, don't panic. This is one of several treatment options for postpartum depression and it is not your only choice. The good news is that if you decide to take an antidepressant for your PPD, you can still benefit greatly from the natural therapies in this book.

Keeping your doctor in the loop is also important because he or she may be able to diagnose physical causes for some of the symptoms you're experiencing. In addition, your doctor is trained to see the big picture and how all of the changes you have already undergone may have added up to trigger the PPD you're experiencing. Your doctor can also evaluate how the steps you are looking at taking to combat the depression may work—or not work—together.

The Edinburgh Postnatal Depression Scale*

Instructions: To correctly take this postpartum depression test, please select the answer which comes closest to how you have felt during the past seven days only—not just how you feel today.

Answer the following ten questions by choosing the appropriate response. You can take the completed test to your doctor for evaluation.

During The Past 7 Days:

1. I have been able to laugh and see the funny side of things.

    a. As much as I always could

    b. Not quite so much now

    c. Definitely not so much now

    d. Not at all

2. I have looked forward with enjoyment to things.

    a. As much as I ever did

    b. Rather less than I used to

    c. Definitely less than I used to

    d. Hardly at all

3. I have blamed myself unnecessarily when things went wrong.

    a. Yes, most of the time

    b. Yes, some of the time

    c. Not very often

    d. No, never

4. I have been anxious or worried for no good reason.

    a. No, not at all

    b. Hardly ever

    c. Yes, sometimes

    d. Yes, very often

5. I have felt scared or panicky for no good reason.

   a. Yes, quite a lot

   b. Yes, sometimes

   c. No, not much

   d. No, not at all

6. Things have been getting on top of me.

   a. Yes, most of the time I haven't been able to cope at all

   b. Yes, sometimes I haven't been coping as well as usual

   c. No, most of the time I have coped quite well

   d. No, I have been coping as well as ever

7. I have been so unhappy that I have had difficulty sleeping.

   a. Yes, most of the time

   b. Yes, some of the time

   c. Not very often

   d. No, not at all

8. I have felt sad or miserable.

   a. Yes, most of the time

   b. Yes, some of the time

   c. Not very often

   d. No, not at all

9. I have been so unhappy that I have been crying.

    a. Yes, most of the time

    b. Yes, quite often

    c. Only occasionally

    d. No, never

10. The thought of harming myself has occurred to me.

a. Yes, quite often

    b. Sometimes

    c. Hardly ever

    d. Never

*Source: J.L. Cox, J.M. Holden, and R. Sagovsky, "Detection of Postnatal Depression: Development of the 10-item Edinburgh Postnatal Depression Scale," *British Journal of Psychiatry* 150 (1987): 782-86.

CHAPTER 7

Healthy Diet—You're Still Eating for Two

Let food be thy medicine and medicine be thy food.

~ HIPPOCRATES

When you were pregnant, there's a good chance food was frequently on your mind and often a topic of conversation. Between cravings and aversions, trying to gain healthy baby weight while not gaining too much excess weight, food was probably a major consideration. Then there's what everyone else thought—friends and family probably differed wildly, some urging seconds on you, others convinced you should watch every bite, and your doctor probably had another set of guidelines altogether.

And the biggest consideration was that you were eating for two. Whatever you ate, your baby essentially ate. Getting the right nutrients was crucial. As was getting enough calories, since a healthy body weight is one of the prerequisites of a healthy birth.

So now you've had the baby. Whew! All that's over, right?

Well, not quite. You're still eating for two, even though you've had your baby. If you're breastfeeding, what you eat can still affect your baby as it is passed on through the breast milk. But the other way what you eat can impact your baby is by how the food you eat affects you.

Why Your Diet Is Important

When you're already battling depression, it may be hard to care about everyday life, about preparing a nutritious meal and sitting down to eat it. In addition, if the introduction of a new baby into the household has caused routines to dissolve into chaos, and no one is handling the responsibility of grocery shopping and there's nothing worth eating in the house, it is that much harder to avoid the fast food trap or the eat-whatever-is-available diet. Last, depression can play havoc with your appetite, sending it in either direction; some people overeat in an attempt to stop the depression or "feed" the feeling, while others find themselves nauseated at the sight of food, unable to find anything that's remotely palatable no matter how hungry they become.

Your diet is important for a number of reasons. Medical researchers believe there's a link between a junk food diet and a risk of depression. If you are already depressed, you don't want to stress your body further by eating unhealthy foods.

A healthy diet is important if you're suffering from PPD because it can keep your blood sugar levels balanced as well as help you avoid cravings.

When it comes to defining a healthy diet, the basics have not changed significantly from what you probably learned growing up. You need to eat a balanced meal, taking in protein, complex carbohydrates and a limited number of fats. You should try to get the recommended 64 ounces of water every day (soda doesn't count), as well as several servings of fruit and vegetables. Choose foods that are high in protein and low in fat, and choose complex carbohydrates (whole grain) over simple (refined white flour, refined sugar).

Foods to Eat and Why

Eating a healthy diet while eating on the run can be a challenge. You can simplify the process by identifying which healthy food groups are the best to choose meals and snacks from. Sometimes limiting your options makes it easier to decide on something healthy so you actually sit down and eat the meal. After all, not every meal has to be a work of art, or even a sit-down affair. It just needs to be healthy, complete and actually consumed—skipping meals isn't healthy, especially if you're breastfeeding.

Protein

Protein provides the body with the amino acids that are the building blocks of healthy tissues and muscles. Protein helps carry nutrients through the body and helps build lean muscle tissue, which can help you lose weight. The more lean body mass you have, the more efficiently you can burn fat.

Protein is also important to a new mother battling PPD because it is an essential part of the production and regulation of hormones in women who are pregnant or have recently given birth. Hormonal changes are one theory behind the causes of postpartum depression, so eating right to help balance hormones just makes good sense.

Some healthy sources of protein include:

- Lean meats, like fish, chicken or other poultry
- Lentils and peas
- Beans
- Nuts

Complex Carbohydrates

Carbohydrates have gotten bad press for many years, but the so-called "good carbs," or complex carbohydrates, are essential to a healthy diet. Complex carbohydrates such as whole grains, legumes, leafy vegetables and fruit can fuel your energy and can also raise your serotonin levels. Because serotonin is one of the neurotransmitters that helps improve mood, and that may be out of balance in the brain during depression, it is important not to rule out carbs just because you want to lose the baby weight faster. Just pick and be choosy, looking for high quality, complex carbohydrates such as:

- Sweet potatoes
- Green vegetables
- Legumes
- Whole grains and whole grain bread

While corn and potatoes fall into both the easy-to-prepare and tasty categories, when you're looking for complex carbs, these two vegetables don't quite measure up with the others. A potato has nutritional value, but it is also a very starchy food, and corn has very little value to back up its taste. For a rounded diet, your vegetable choices should ensure full value of nutrients and fiber.

Fiber

Fiber helps the body keep the digestive system in good shape, so you're not dealing with either diarrhea or constipation while taking on the responsibilities of new motherhood. Fiber can also help energize the body by correcting the speed of digestion and giving the body a chance to utilize the nutrients from other foods.

Some foods rich in fiber include:

- Whole wheat pastas
- Whole grains such as barley, corn and brown rice
- Broccoli, cauliflower, tomatoes and green peas
- Kidney beans, lima beans, chick peas and lentils

Fats

Fat was once considered the culprit in all weight gain, but in recent years medical science has come to understand that simple carbohydrates are far more likely to pack on the pounds than fat. That said, fat does have nine calories per gram whereas carbohydrates have four, and complex carbs are good for you.

Fats can also be good for you—at least, some of them. For overall heart health, it is no surprise that you should avoid or limit butter, cream cheese, creamers, bacon, sour cream, fatty cheeses and possibly red meat. Some of the healthier fats include olives and olive oil, peanuts and peanut butter, almonds, avocados and sesame seeds.

Omega-3 essential fatty acids are important to your diet. These essential fatty acids cannot be manufactured by the body and must be consumed through diet. Fish is a great source of omega-3 fatty acids; these amino acids can be found in tuna, salmon, halibut, other seafood including algae, and in some plants and nuts. If you would rather avoid seafood because of a concern for methyl/mercury found in fish, there are many good supplements you can take, including those from krill oil. The benefits of these supplements are the same as fish oil.

Medical studies on omega-3 fatty acids and depression have shown varied results, with many studies indicating that including the essential fatty acids in diet can help combat depression. Other studies have shown that omega-3 fatty acids in conjunction with antidepressants can help where depression is concerned. According to the website MayoClinic.com, some of those studies have shown that including omega-3 fatty acids in one's diet, or correcting a deficiency of the acids, can help protect against postpartum depression.

In addition to possible positive effects on depression, omega-3 fatty acids may help lower the risk of heart disease, some cancers and arthritis. They may also be important for brain function, memory and behavioral function, as they are concentrated in the brain. Infants need to receive omega-3 fatty acids from their mothers to help avoid vision and nerve problems.

If your diet is deficient in omega-3 fatty acids, you may exhibit symptoms including dry and flaking skin, poor memory, poor circulation, heart problems and memory problems.

Hydration—Water and Green Tea

You need to drink adequate fluids all the time, not just when pregnant, breastfeeding or battling postpartum depression. And drinking enough water may not increase your breast milk, but not drinking enough can affect the amount you have.

Soda is a bad choice when you're dealing with postpartum depression—you are better off without the boost, peak and crash of a sugared, caffeinated beverage. Water does a great job at hydrating, without the sugar or artificial sweeteners that sodas contain.

Green tea is another really good choice for hydration. Green tea is a powerful antioxidant, one of the food sources in a group called catechins, which help halt oxidative damage to cells and promote health. Green tea can reduce your risk of

- Heart disease
- Bladder cancer
- Esophageal colon and lung cancers
- Breast cancer and skin cancer

Green tea can also help block the bad cholesterol (LDL) while increasing good (HDL) cholesterol levels. As long as you're eating and drinking for two, you might as well plan ahead for a healthy future, too.

Increasing your water or green tea consumption can help you lose weight, in part by flushing out bloating, and in part because you feel full sooner when you're drinking as much water as you're eating. Green tea will also take the place of other, more caloric foods and beverages that you would otherwise consume. Additionally, clinical studies have shown that the fat-burning effect of green tea and caffeine may be due in part to the catechins in the tea.

Green tea is also a good choice because it is much lower in caffeine than black teas and is generally regarded as a more calming drink than, say, a cup of coffee.

Foods to Avoid and Why

Along with a balanced diet of healthy foods, there are some foods and beverages that are best avoided.

Sugar is a quick fix of energy, but it wears off much too fast, making blood sugar levels spike with a quick, false energy that soon drops and leaves you feeling even more enervated and exhausted than before.

Sugar can cause an artificial mood swing, making you feel as if you're happier—until the body processes the sugar and you're faced with the post-sugar crash. That's why those of us who suffer from Seasonal Affective Disorder (SAD), seasonal depression caused by the low light of winter months, crave simple carbs; we want that rush of sugar, the blood sugar spike, and that transitory happiness. Unfortunately for the new mom battling postpartum depression, the quick fix ends with a lower low and even less energy. If you feel you can't give up sugar, at least try to cut down.

The same goes for caffeine. The quick fix of caffeine is a bad idea for a nursing mom, with the same jolt of energy followed by a crash. In addition, both sugar and caffeine can increase the jittery, anxious feelings that a new mom battling PPD may already be fighting. And if you're breastfeeding, your baby is also getting caffeine, which might make it harder for your child to sleep at a time when you both may badly need the sleep.

If you're not nursing, abstaining from alcohol may not seem necessary any longer. Although it may be true that a glass of wine with dinner won't hurt, keep in mind that alcohol is a depressant. For a woman fighting postpartum depression, adding a depressant into your system is counter-productive. In addition, while initially alcohol might make you sleepy, it tends to interrupt sleep and lead to a poor quality of sleep overall (see *Chapter 17: Rest Up—A Guide for Sleep*).

Meal Portions and Frequency

A Zen koan (or parable) reads, "When you are hungry, eat; when you are tired, sleep." Unfortunately, for many of us in western civilization, being sleep deprived, hungry, and on the run seem to go together.

Some studies suggest that a new mom should eat every two to three hours throughout the day rather than relying on the standard three-meals-a-day tradition. The idea is to eat smaller meals to make sure you're not becoming overly hungry and overeating, and to make certain you're refueling adequately, given all the new responsibilities in your life. Some guidelines state that you should be eating approximately 1,500 to 1,800 calories a day if you are breastfeeding, but the exact caloric level that works for you according to your energy levels, daily physical demands, and body size is a guideline best determined with your doctor.

You should avoid eating within three hours of going to bed for the night. Give yourself time to digest before you try to sleep—you will get better nutrient value from your food and better quality sleep. Additionally, you should try to eat at regular times, making good, healthy choices. If you can fall into a routine, finding the time to eat might not be quite so difficult. Choose healthy snack foods—a handful of nuts, a bunch of grapes, an apple, some whole wheat snack crackers and cheese. Eating a healthy diet is good for you physically and mentally during this busy time when you're still eating for two.

CHAPTER 8

Pregnancy, Hormones and Depression

I am only one, but I am one. I cannot do everything, but I can do something. And I will not let what I cannot do interfere with what I can do.

~ EDWARD EVERETT HALE

P regnancy changes hormone levels throughout your body. Some researchers believe that a sudden drop in hormones that occurs right after giving birth can trigger postpartum depression. Levels of thyroid hormones may also drop after giving birth. Thyroid hormones regulate how the body stores and releases caloric energy from food, and low thyroid can cause depression.

What's Going on in Your Body

In less politically correct times, it was common to attribute any mood swings a pregnant woman or new mom experienced to hormones. It was also common to treat this lightly, as if mood and emotional swings were simply part of being female.

Hormones do affect mood, and hormones unique to women can lead to depression, even without the physical and emotional stress of pregnancy, birth and caring for a new child.

During pregnancy, levels of naturally occurring steroid hormones, estrogen and progesterone, rise in your body. After you've given birth, those levels drop back to normal levels very quickly, and some research suggests this sudden rise and drop of hormones can trigger postpartum depression much the same way smaller rises and drops during the menstrual cycle can produce PMS.

Hormones directly affect the brain chemistry that controls emotions. Uniquely female hormones that rise during pregnancy and drop during birth can disrupt the normal functioning of neurotransmitters such as serotonin, which carry messages from the brain to the nervous system and which have a direct impact on mood (many western medicine antidepressant drugs work directly on serotonin—how it's released and reabsorbed by the brain).

Thyroid hormones can also drop after birth. The thyroid is a small gland in the throat that helps the body determine how best to use and burn calories. Hypothyroidism is a physical disorder where the thyroid underperforms and can lead to weight gain, lethargy, and depression. Low levels of thyroid after giving birth have been theorized to be one of the causes of PPD.

Natural Solutions for Hormone Regulation

One of the natural solutions to regulating female hormones is exercise. Regular exercise can help keep your stress hormones—cortisol and adrenaline—in check. Head out the door for a brisk 30-minute walk and you'll flush a lot of those anxiety-producing chemicals out of your body. Anxiety is often one of the symptoms of postpartum depression.

Exercise can also help balance your estrogen and progesterone levels that soared during pregnancy and then dropped. Finding the right balance for these hormones can significantly improve mood, especially as these hormones can disrupt the function of neurotransmitters such as serotonin. Regulating hormones through exercise is a great benefit for breastfeeding moms who don't want to take medications. For an added benefit, exercising can help you start shedding the baby weight, which makes most moms feel better about themselves.

Setting your body in motion can also trigger other hormones. Exercise causes the brain to release endorphins, sometimes called natural opiates. Endorphins are a group of hormones known as peptides. Secreted in the brain and nervous system, they are known to have an analgesic (painkilling) effect and are considered "feel good" hormones.

Herbal Options

Natural and alternative medicine offers herbal remedies for PPD. Among those, Vitex Agnus-castus, fruit of the chaste tree, is used for irregularities of menstrual cycles, for PMS and for regulating progesterone. Motherwort and lemon balm can help stabilize mood swings and bring emotions back into balance. For more information on herbal solutions to postpartum depression, see *Chapter 9: Vitamins, Minerals, Herbal Supplements and Food.*

Acupuncture

Acupuncture is an ancient Chinese medical practice that treats the entire body and spirit holistically through the use of needles placed in the skin at specific stimulation points on the body. Acupuncture treats PPD through techniques that increase energy, strengthen the immune system, and balance hormones. In addition to needlework, this method addresses postpartum depression by focusing on nutrients the mother may have depleted while giving birth. For more on acupuncture and postpartum depression, see *Chapter 12: Take a Break—Relaxation and Stress Management.*

Traditional Chinese Medicine

Traditional Chinese Medicine views the heart as the center for the spirit and mind and for regulating blood. If PPD has resulted from blood loss during birth, the "spirit-mind," as it's referred to by its practitioners, may be undernourished and restless, which can result in depression symptoms. Traditional Chinese Medicine goes on to describe symptoms of fatigue, anxiety, mood swings, guilt, reduced breast milk supply and even heart palpitations, all resulting from the spirit-mind being out of balance.

This branch of medicine, considered alternative in the U.S., is over 3,000 years old and combines herbal medicines, massage, acupuncture, exercise and food therapy to balance the yin and yang forces in the body.

Hormone Therapy

Hormone replacement therapy uses supplemental estrogen, typically synthetic, to counteract the drop in the hormone at birth and regulate levels in the body. It is not always effective and there is limited research on it at this time. Hormone replacement therapy can take the form of pills, injections or skin patches. A blood test can identify whether hormone levels are out of balance enough to warrant replacement therapy.

Hormone replacement therapy is not recommended for breastfeeding moms, though breastfeeding itself can become therapeutic for mothers struggling with PPD. In addition, hormone therapy can decrease milk production, another reason to look at natural solutions.

A more natural solution exists today. Bioidentical hormones are used in hormone replacement therapy (HRT) with menopausal women and can also be useful in treating PMS and PPD. Bioidentical hormones are created from natural sources, wild yam and soy beans, and match exactly the hormones your body produces. Because of the match, the body metabolizes bioidentical hormones as if it had produced them itself and there are far fewer side effects than traditional HRT. Some of the bioidentical hormones include 17 beta-estradiol, estrone and estriol. The bioidentical version of progesterone is simply progesterone created for better absorption. The bioidentical supplements come in many forms, including sublingual (under the tongue), pill, patch, and creams.

Bioidentical estrogen has been effectively used for women suffering panic attacks and nervousness due to menopausal reduction of natural estrogen. Studies in both the Journal of Clinical Psychiatry and Lancet have shown that bioidentical estrogen can effectively treat postpartum depression. In the first study, 83 percent of the 23 women receiving bioidentical hormone showed clinical recovery by the second week of treatment.

Bioidentical hormones are a more natural choice for treating postpartum depression than antidepressants, which don't actually affect the hormone levels of the body but work instead on neurotransmitters. They are also more natural than hormone replacement therapies. However, a prescription is required and you should talk to your doctor before embarking on any kind of hormone regulating therapy, including natural therapies such as herbal solutions. If you are breastfeeding, make sure you have all the information before you make your decision.

CHAPTER 9

Vitamins, Minerals, Herbal Supplements and Food

There is a proper balance between not asking enough of oneself and asking or expecting too much.

~ MAY SARTON

Pregnancy and birth are hard on a woman's body. Stress and hormone levels increase considerably through pregnancy and drop during labor, and thyroid function can decrease after giving birth.

Postpartum depression can add a host of physical problems that creep in, from fatigue to sleeplessness. Breastfeeding continues drawing nutrients from the mother's body to support the child, the same way the mother's body played host and supplied all needed nutrients and building blocks during the pregnancy. In the case of a difficult birth, especially one where there is significant maternal blood loss, the mother is depleted at a time when she needs all her energy to enjoy her new life with her new baby.

For the last nine months before the birth, the mother's body has treated the baby as the number one concern. Nutrients and supplements that the baby needed were received from the mother. So if you started off deficient in some nutrient, you are probably even more deficient in it now.

Depleting

Some of the deficiencies you may be facing postpartum include zinc, one of the minerals required for cell division and therefore one of the minerals the baby needs to take from the mother during pregnancy. After birth, many mothers have low levels of zinc, which has been linked to postpartum depression.

B vitamins are essential for energy, but they also play a part in regulating the hormones estrogen and progesterone, which increase levels in the body rapidly during pregnancy and then go back to normal directly after the birth. B vitamins can help you regulate these hormones again and may help alleviate symptoms of PPD.

Feeling a little hazy and confused? Pregnancy and birth also deplete your stores of omega-3 fatty acids, which are essential to the proper functioning of the brain and nervous system. During pregnancy the baby needs EPA and DHA, the long-chain omega-3 fatty acids, as its nervous system develops, and the mother's body diverts her supply of the fatty acids for the child's development.

After birth, the child continues to need the fatty acids for ongoing development. One study showed that omega-3s in breast milk don't come from the mother's current diet but from the mother's reserves, so if you're going to supplement, starting before breastfeeding begins is a good idea. Studies have shown that supplementing with omega-3 fatty acids will have a benefit to the child who receives the nutrients through breast milk.

Keep in mind that *you* need omega-3 fatty acids, too. One study in 2002 showed that women who ate high levels of seafood while pregnant had higher levels of DHA in their milk after birth and had lower incidences of postpartum depression.

Adrenal glands are also hard hit by the pregnancy and birth cycle. Adrenals provide reserves of strength during the stress of pregnancy and delivery and the lack of sleep after the birth. Depleted adrenal glands can cause hormonal problems.

If the birth was accompanied by blood loss, you may be deficient in calcium and magnesium, which need to remain in balance with each other. Calcium helps blood coagulate and magnesium helps muscles relax. Midwives are said to use calcium-rich herbs and plants to assist labor and postpartum recovery. Calcium can of course be supplemented and is also found in foods including yogurt, sesame seeds, dairy products, dark leafy vegetables and blackstrap molasses (which is also a great source of iron).

Calcium is also needed to start rebuilding bone density after birth. During pregnancy the fetus absorbs needed calcium directly from the mother, depleting her supply. The combination of calcium, magnesium and zinc in a supplement aids in the absorption and use of each mineral in the body. Breastfeeding mothers can supplement but should inform their doctors.

Vitamin K can also help rebuild iron stores after blood loss. It can be found in those same leafy greens the calcium comes from, and in the mother's breast milk it can help prevent the baby from having a deficiency of the vitamin.

Rebuilding

Fortunately, there are steps you can take to help replenish your body naturally, using vitamins and herbal supplements. Many of these natural solutions can help with depression, anxiety, mental clarity, sleep, energy and libido, as well as get you back on your feet and improve breastfeeding.

Before starting any kind of supplementation, you should keep your primary care doctor or ob/gyn in the loop. Take a list of all medications and over-the-counter products you may be taking (including any vitamins you're currently taking) and explain what you'd like to try and why. Your doctor can help you sort out whether or not there could be any interactions between the vitamins, herbs and supplements you want to try, whether there are any known side effects and whether there could be any concern taking them if you are breastfeeding. For the most part, natural supplements and vitamins have far fewer side effects than pharmaceuticals but you will want to have all the facts before you put anything new into your body.

One supplement that has been shown to have a positive effect on postpartum depression is SAMe, S-Adenosyl-L-Methionine, a substance that occurs naturally in the body's cells and is derived from amino acids (found naturally in protein-rich foods). SAMe is part of the processes that regulate serotonin, melatonin, dopamine, and adrenaline, as well as neurotransmitters. Supplementation with SAMe can help combat PPD. However, results from placebo tests with SAMe don't show consistent results of improvement of postpartum depression symptoms, and SAMe is not recommended for breastfeeding mothers due to a lack of evidence of its effects.

Herbs

Herbs have been used in medicines for at least 3,000 years by Asian, African and indigenous American cultures. Some 80 percent of people in the world still use herbal remedies for some or all of their healthcare needs. Even today's pharmaceuticals evolved in some manner from traditional medicines, though they are very far removed from original herbal medicines.

Herbs can be used for a variety of physical and emotional ailments, including symptoms of postpartum depression such as depression, anxiety, lack of mental clarity, hormonal imbalances, sleep disturbances, low energy and low libido. Herbal remedies are usually made up of stems, leaves, flowers and seeds of plants that can be taken as teas, tinctures, capsules and powders.

Not every herbal solution is appropriate for a breastfeeding mother, and some herbal remedies can even cause side effects. Quality control has also been an issue. In June 2010, the United States Food and Drug Administration (FDA) began requiring companies that manufacture herbal supplements to follow strict quality manufacturing standards. However, inspections of the plants are few and far between. Thus, be cautious in selecting only high quality herbal supplements and take notice of any reactions as you use them.

The following are herbs that may be helpful in relieving symptoms of postpartum depression:

St. John's Wort is often used to treat depression. It is a natural antidepressant and has antibacterial, anti-inflammatory, anti-viral and pain-relieving properties. It can be more effective than pharmaceutical antidepressants. It is considered safe for breastfeeding mothers, but let your doctor know before you start. There are some medications that St. John's Wort should not be taken in conjunction with, including oral contraceptives, which become less effective. St. John's Wort can also cause some side effects, including dizziness, confusion, tiredness and sedation.

Motherwort and **lemon balm** can help control mood swings.

Skullcap and **chamomile** help ease feelings of stress and nervous anxiety.

Vitex Agnus-Castus is sometimes referred to as the "woman's herb" because it works so well with women's bodies; essentially, this herb works to regulate female hormones. The fruit and seed of the chaste tree, Vitex can be used to treat PMS and menstrual irregularities and to prevent miscarriages. After birth it can help control bleeding and increase production of breast milk. Vitex can also help with nervousness, joint conditions, headaches, body inflammation and swelling.

Valerian is debated somewhat as a natural sleep aid. Though it is thought to be safe, it is not recommended for use by pregnant or breastfeeding mothers. The herb, taken as a supplement, sometimes works better after several weeks' use. In addition, it is apt to cause side effects such as headache, dizziness, stomach upset and sleeplessness, which is the very thing you are trying to correct. In addition, valerian may interact with prescription drugs and alcohol. You may be better off with a cup of chamomile tea.

Gingko Biloba is one of the best-known herbs, touted for aiding mental clarity and depression. In addition, according to

Discovery Health, gingko biloba increases blood flow to both the brain and the sexual organs, which can increase sexual desire in both men and women, and enhance orgasm. It is natural for a woman's libido to dip after childbirth even without the complications of postpartum depression. A natural boost in the direction of enhanced libido couldn't hurt.

Even though herbs have been in use for at least 3,000 years and probably longer, before starting any new supplementation program, talk to your doctor, especially if you're breastfeeding.

Nourishing Your Way Through Depression

Studies have shown that people dealing with mood disorders and depression such as PPD are less apt to eat healthy, regular meals. Yet to beat postpartum depression, you will need essential vitamin and minerals that are present in healthy foods and supplements.

Nutrients are what our bodies are made of. We use carbohydrates for energy, proteins to create muscle, and various vitamins and minerals for cellular processes. There are foods that can promote sleep and those that can change your mood, and for the most part as a new mom, you need to eat a well-rounded diet. By including a little bit of everything—proteins, fats, complex carbohydrates—you can replenish your body so that you can continue to fight postpartum depression.

Antioxidants

Antioxidants are molecules that inhibit the breakdown of free radicals, which are damaging molecules that are produced naturally and cause aging and bodily dysfunction. A good multivitamin will likely provide you with your antioxidants on a daily basis, but you can supplement with food choices that not only boost your mood but also help you combat postpartum depression.

You can reduce the effect of free radicals on your body and battle PPD by including foods rich in antioxidants such as beta-carotene, vitamin C and vitamin E. Good food sources of these antioxidants are:

- Beta-carotene: apricots, broccoli, grapefruit, carrots, collards, peaches, pumpkin, spinach, sweet potatoes.

- Vitamin C: blueberries, broccoli, grapefruit, kiwi, oranges, peppers, potatoes, tomatoes.

- Vitamin E: nuts, seeds, vegetable oils, wheat germ.

Proteins

Protein-rich foods contain tyrosine, an amino acid that has a positive effect on the neurotransmitters dopamine and norepinephrine, which directly impact mood. Great sources for lean proteins include turkey, tuna and chicken. Breastfeeding moms may want to watch the amount of fish they consume due to mercury levels. Some low-mercury fish options include Tilapia, shrimp, salmon and cod. Other sources include dairy products, cheese, eggs, lean meats, fish, yogurt, beans and peas.

Carbs

Carbohydrates have gotten a bad rap for many years because medical research has shown that excess carbs turn to sugar in the body and sugar stores itself as fat. But there are good carbs and bad carbs. Bad carbs are refined sugars and flours, junk food, sweets, candy and many baked goods. Good carbohydrate choices include whole grains, fruits, vegetables and legumes.

Vitamins

Studies have shown that many people with depression have vitamin D deficiencies. You can supplement your vitamin D, you can head outside into the sun, and you can include some of the following foods in your diet: swordfish, tuna, salmon, fortified orange juice, milk, yogurt, sardines, beef, eggs, fortified cereals and various cheeses.

Folic acid, part of the B-vitamin complex, can be depleted during pregnancy and that depletion causes depression-like symptoms: insomnia, forgetfulness, anxiety, irritability and lethargy. Though vitamin B deficiency has not been causally connected to postpartum depression, vitamin B is good for converting amino acids into the neurotransmitters that effect mood, serotonin and norepinephrine. According to MayoClinic.com, B-complex vitamins or supplements of B6 and B12 are considered "likely safe" for use while breastfeeding when used in normal daily dosages and not long term.

Minerals

One mineral that can aid in beating depression is selenium. Selenium supplementation should be limited because dosages higher than recommended levels can be toxic. If you limit your intake to food sources of selenium, it is hard to overdose because naturally occurring quantities are relatively small. Foods rich in selenium include beans and legumes, lean meat, dairy products, nuts and seeds, seafood and whole grains.

Omega-3 Fatty Acids

Omega-3 fatty acids are essential fatty acids the body needs in order to maintain health, especially heart health, but which the body cannot produce on its own. Omega-3 fatty acids are said to help improve symptoms of depression and mood swings (see *Chapter 7: Healthy Diet—You're Still Eating for Two*).

Good dietary sources of omega-3 fatty acids are fish (especially salmon, mackerel, halibut, sardines, tuna and herring), flaxseeds and flaxseed oil, walnuts and walnut oil, and dark green leafy vegetables. You can also take an omega-3 fatty acid supplement.

CHAPTER 10

Make Your Move— Exercise and Depression

Movement is a medicine for creating change in a person's physical, emotional, and mental states.

~ CAROL WELCH

The catch-22 of exercise and depression is that the depression itself makes it hard to want to do anything, especially something that takes a lot of energy you don't have, like exercise. Hopefully by knowing that exercise can help you feel more energetic after you've exercised will help motivate you at the outset.

One of the symptoms of depression is a loss of interest in activities you once enjoyed. If you are a runner and ran throughout your pregnancy, having lost the urge to run (or even just the willingness to get up, find your shoes and head out the door) can make you feel like you've lost a part of yourself.

If you were fit before your pregnancy, know that you can get that level of fitness back. It is understandable that having lost ground makes you feel frustrated. Feeling like you're starting over can be daunting. Fortunately, you are not starting from scratch; if you were fit, your muscle memory will help you get back in shape faster than if you hadn't been working out before the pregnancy. If you were involved in a sport or a fitness routine before your pregnancy, getting back to it might help you feel like the old pre-PPD you.

If you were not fit before your pregnancy, this is a great time to think about getting there. You have a new baby in your life to take care of, and that means taking care of yourself, too.

Exercise can help fight depression because it feels like you're actually doing something—as you are—to physically combat the depression. Taking steps can make you feel better, and when you start seeing progress both in your fitness levels and in how you're feeling emotionally, both will give you another mental boost.

If exercise sounds like a chore and something that's going to isolate you even more, find a way around that barrier. Some forms of exercise are social—go take a spinning class, look for a runners' group, or find an amateur team sport in your community. If you're comfortable joining a gym, you can be around people even if you're shy and don't want to interact. Just being around other people who are engaged in doing something physical can improve your mood. And sometimes seeing what others in the gym are achieving can help you create manageable goals. Once you start going regularly and seeing some of the same friendly faces, you'll not only be more comfortable and have a sense of community, you'll have people who are expecting you and charting your progress even if you're not.

Exercise burns up stress chemicals. Stress causes the body to produce adrenaline and other fight or flight chemicals even when you're not facing an actual emergency. If you are constantly poised for emergency action that never comes, the stress chemicals like adrenaline and cortisol (which is often present in the body when someone is depressed, and which is already present in elevated levels in the body after the birth of a child) can wear down the body and put a strain on the immune system.

Exercise also interrupts your train of thought. It is hard to keep the same anxious or obsessive thought pattern going when you are putting a lot of concentration into running or rowing or participating in a team sport. Interrupting the obsessive, anxious or depressive thoughts can derail them and rob them of their power over you.

After you have worked out, the chemicals released in your body—neurotransmitters and endorphins—make you feel more confident. That positive outlook makes it harder for the depression to return right away. Working out will also raise your body temperature, which can be calming.

Exercise does not have to be all or nothing, and it does not have to be all at once. For the best benefit to boosting mood and promoting weight loss and fitness, at least 30 minutes a day, three to five days a week seems to be the gold standard. But if that is hard to fit in to the new schedule with the new baby, it should be reassuring to know that a little is better than nothing. There are positive effects to be gained from whatever level of movement you can add to your day. Want to put on some music and dance through the living room with the baby? You can bond with your new child while you're moving and releasing stress chemicals and flooding your body with healthy chemicals. There are many ways to add movement to your day—take the stairs rather than an elevator, walk the escalator rather than riding, park farther away, and walk to short errands.

Short may be sweet, but consistency counts. Those people who maintain an exercise routine will see more results than those who are hit or miss. The more months you work out, the greater the cumulative effect on your emotional health.

What and Where

You don't have to join a gym and go sweat among grunting bodybuilders if that's not your thing. If there is something you love to do, finding a way to do it can help improve your mood just by doing it.

If you don't have anything you love to do exercise-wise, find something you don't hate. Millions of New Year's Resolutions are abandoned every March (or earlier) because people assumed that being healthy and working out had to be loathsome experiences. If you like walking, take walks. Ask friends to join you for company. A walking buddy can keep you on schedule even if it's not the nicest day outside and you'd rather stay in. Take your baby in a baby pack and spend some quality bonding time together.

Whatever you love to do, if you can find a way to do it consistently, the rewards will be greater than whatever effort you had to put out to get to the work out.

Sneak It In

Just as working out doesn't have to mean getting dressed and going to a gym, working out doesn't have to be "official." Anytime you can add movement to your day, you can boost your mood and benefit your body. Whether you're working or at home, look for ways to sneak some physical activity into your day.

- Park farther away from wherever you're going (doctor's office, work, the grocery store)

- Walk on a treadmill or in place when you're on the phone

- Go outside to play with your children rather than playing video games or watching TV

- Start a buddy system—exercise buddies can keep you going

- Try something new for fun—a dance class, yoga, bike riding

- Clean house—aggressively!

- When you stand up, stretch

A Physical Activity chart is included in the appendix of this book to help you track your exercise.

CHAPTER 11

Hypnosis—Using the Power of Your Mind

Whatever we plant in our subconscious mind and nourish with repetition and emotion will one day become a reality.

~ EARL NIGHTINGALE

As a certified hypnotherapist in private practice, I have worked with thousands of clients on a vast number of issues, including depression, anxiety, stress, insomnia, low self-esteem, fear, and various physical symptoms of pain. I have had the pleasure of witnessing dramatic results in very short periods of time.

Oftentimes when people first contemplate using hypnosis for their issues, they feel unsure or apprehensive. By and large, this is because of numerous misconceptions of hypnosis perpetuated by stage hypnotists and the portrayal of hypnosis in the entertainment and media industries. Entertainment has its value, but clinical hypnosis (also known as therapeutic hypnosis) is in a different class and has a completely different purpose.

Fortunately, there has been a growing awareness of clinical hypnosis in the press. With more and more people choosing to follow an integrative, holistic, mind-body approach to medical and psychological healing, hypnosis is gaining renewed interest and appreciation.

Because of the profound results I have not only witnessed, but experienced personally, I know that hypnosis is an extremely useful natural therapy that you can use to help combat postpartum depression and other postpartum issues. I will discuss the use of both hypnosis and subliminal music recordings and explain each in more detail. Each method has its place, and you will learn more about both later in this chapter.

This chapter will explain what hypnosis is—and is not—and will explore the power of the subconscious mind on our attitudes, beliefs, behaviors and feelings. It will also describe the effectiveness of self-hypnosis, hypnotherapy, and hypnosis and subliminal recordings in bringing remarkable change to your life.

Common Misconceptions—What Hypnosis Is Not

Hypnosis is still truly misunderstood by many, and because it is misunderstood, it is therefore often met with fear. This is a shame, since hypnosis is such a powerful tool that almost anyone can use at any time, wherever one is, to make positive changes to one's life. We will get into the details of how to use this tool to your benefit further on, but first and foremost, it is important to explore the common misconceptions.

1. **When a person is hypnotized, he/she is asleep or unconscious**

   This is one of the most widely held misconceptions about hypnosis because people who are hypnotized often have their eyes closed and remain very still. While hypnotized, a person is often deeply and profoundly relaxed, but at the same time, they are alert and highly focused. No one ever loses consciousness under hypnosis. On occasion, a person may become so relaxed that they drift into sleep.

2. **A person can be hypnotized against his/her will and can be made to do anything**

   No one can be forced into hypnosis. If a person does not want to be hypnotized, it won't happen. Nor can one be made to do anything one does not want to do while under hypnosis. If a suggestion were ever given that was disagreeable, one's subconscious would simply not accept it.

3. **While under hypnosis, a person will divulge deep, personal secrets**

   Although typically very relaxed, a person who is hypnotized is also aware and in control the entire time. The choice is his/hers whether to share a secret or not to share a secret.

4. **Not everyone can be hypnotized—only the weak-minded, gullible or stupid**
   Almost anyone of at least average intelligence can be hypnotized, as long as they want to be hypnotized and have the ability to focus, concentrate, and follow direction. Bright, creative-minded people tend to do the best under hypnosis.

5. **People can get stuck in hypnosis**
   No one has ever gotten stuck in hypnosis. The only reason a person would remain in hypnosis is that they choose to, because it is such a comfortable state. Many of my clients tell me the only thing about the session they don't like is ending the hypnosis because it feels so good.

Facts—What Hypnosis Is

Hypnosis is a safe, side effect-free way to effectively and positively influence your health, both emotionally and physically. According to medical research, hypnosis is believed to help relieve depression when used to treat symptoms of depression. Hypnosis has been used in the treatment of pain, depression, anxiety, stress, compulsive behavior, and many other psychological and medical problems.

Hypnosis is a relaxed, focused state of concentration. During hypnosis, your focus, concentration and inner absorption is heightened, while distractions are blocked out. The analytical (rational), conscious mind relaxes, and the subconscious mind becomes more receptive to positive suggestions and affirmations for reaching your desired goals. In essence, hypnosis is a means of communication between the conscious and subconscious mind. In order to understand why this communication is important, we need to understand how the subconscious mind and conscious mind work, and how they differ.

We all have two layers of consciousness—the conscious mind and the subconscious mind. All of the memories, feelings, and emotions from everything we have ever experienced are stored within the subconscious mind. While we may not have conscious memory of those experiences, our subconscious mind stores that information to develop our core beliefs, behaviors and habits.

The conscious mind is the analytical, rational part of our mind. The conscious mind processes and analyzes information from what we experience to determine whether the information supports the beliefs and behavioral patterns already stored in our subconscious mind. If the existing beliefs are supported, the conscious mind allows this information to move into the subconscious mind to build upon those pre-existing beliefs.

During hypnosis, in addition to being more receptive to positive suggestions and affirmations, we can also communicate directly with our subconscious mind so habits or beliefs that we have outgrown or no longer serve us can be identified and released. We can then identify our authentic motivations—fears, hopes, and dreams—that are held by the subconscious, and make effective, permanent changes.

Hypnotherapy—Private Hypnosis Sessions

Using the services of a professional, certified hypnotherapist in a private session has many advantages. First, the hypnotherapist is focused on you and only you. Although many people have similar issues, like smoking, weight issues, motivation, or insomnia, the hypnotherapist may decide that for you, your personality, goals, and any other factors he/she deems relevant, one specific method of hypnosis may be more effective than another. In addition, private sessions are just that—private. In the comfort and safety of a room with only you and your hypnotherapist, you can really let go of worries, concerns, tension and stress, and move into deep relaxation.

So how does a private session work? Typically, you would begin by discussing your challenges and goals and what you would like to accomplish using hypnosis. The hypnotherapist will ask all of the necessary questions regarding your issues and aims for the session and will explain hypnosis to you. At the start of the actual hypnosis, the hypnotherapist will often play relaxing music in the background, provide you a comfortable chair in which to recline, possibly dim the lights for comfort, and then guide you into a relaxed state with what is called an induction (to induce relaxation). After the induction, the hypnotherapist has a variety of methods at his or her disposal, including direct suggestion, metaphors, age regression, and emotional release therapy, to name just a few.

Occasionally one session is enough, but typically you may return for one, five, or many more sessions until you and your hypnotherapist feel you have reached your goals. Some hypnotherapists will provide you with a recording of your session or a pre-recorded reinforcement CD.

Self-Hypnosis—The Benefits of Hypnotizing Yourself

Self-hypnosis is a wonderful tool for a new mom to have at her disposal. It is essentially when you hypnotize yourself. Self-hypnosis is often useful as a stress management tool, but you can use it for pretty much any change you want to make. It is more flexible than seeing a hypnotherapist or using recordings, as you do not need to have a hypnotherapist guide you, either personally or by recording.

Similar to meditation, self-hypnosis helps you to relax your body, let stress subside, and distract your mind from unpleasant thoughts or feelings or engage your mind with desired thoughts and feelings. The relaxation achieved through self-hypnosis can be deep. Unlike meditation, positive suggestions or affirmations are added to achieve a specific result. The positive suggestions or affirmations should be worded in a positive manner—"I will" rather than "I won't"—and placed in the immediate future, targeting specific and realistic ends.

Steps for Self-Hypnosis

Here are steps you can take to begin using self-hypnosis. The more you practice self-hypnosis, the easier it will become and the faster you will be able to go into hypnosis.

First, find a place where you will not be disturbed for about 10–12 minutes and get yourself into a relaxed position. You can sit, recline, or lie flat; it doesn't matter, as long as you are comfortable.

Find a spot slightly above eye level and focus your eyes on it. Take a deep breath in, hold it for a moment, and then exhale slowly while allowing your body to relax. Repeat this five times. Imagine your eyes feeling heavier and more relaxed with each deep breath, and feel your body becoming more comfortable and relaxed, as you continue to focus on your deep breathing so that other thoughts and distractions are minimized. Finally, on the fifth deep breath, allow your eyes to close.

Continue to relax your body. You may want to do progressive relaxation, which is to start by focusing on a point on your body, like the top of your head, and slowly move down your body, releasing and relaxing every part of your body, until your whole body has been systematically and progressively relaxed. Or, you may choose to imagine yourself comfortably relaxing in a beautiful, safe place in nature. This can be somewhere you've been before, or a place you have created in your imagination.

Once you feel completely relaxed, select an area of improvement you would like to work on and formulate a positive suggestion or affirmation. Repeat this suggestion to yourself mentally for approximately one minute. (Note: you may find it easier if you select the area of improvement and formulate the suggestions before you begin.)

To end your session, count slowly to yourself from one to five, becoming more alert with each number. Open your eyes on the count of five. Or, if you choose to do self-hypnosis at night before you sleep, count from five to one, keeping your eyes closed and becoming more sleepy with each number, and at the count of one, allow yourself to drift into a comfortable, contented slumber.

Hypnosis Aides

Although it is valuable to have your own personal hypnotherapist guiding you one-on-one in the privacy of an office, you may not have the time, finances or inclination to do so, especially if you are a mom with a newborn to look after. Guided hypnosis recordings are an alternative that are less expensive, less time consuming, totally private, and easy on your schedule. You can listen to them almost anywhere, and whenever you want, and most importantly, with privacy. You can use them repeatedly for as long as you like. I create hypnosis recordings for clients in my practice, and they tell me they love having the recordings on hand, and will pull them out when they need a booster of a session, or when they need to relax or even to help them sleep.

There are important factors to consider when purchasing hypnosis recordings online. One is to be sure that the recordings are made by a qualified, certified hypnotherapist. If the hypnotic suggestions are not given correctly, they can be worthless. Also, you will want the hypnosis recording to cover the specific issues for which you want to make the changes. And third, be sure to listen to a sample of the recording before purchasing. If you find the hypnotherapist's voice annoying, or the music is too loud or not relaxing, or if the recording does not sound professional, you won't benefit the same as you would to a high-quality recording with a soothing voice and pleasing background music.

Subliminal Music

Subliminal music recordings are positive suggestions recorded for the subconscious mind that are below the audible capacity of your conscious mind. With subliminal music recordings, there is no need to consciously relax since the suggestions are inaudible to the conscious mind (thereby surpassing it automatically).

The major benefit to this type of recording is that you can be doing other things without having to stop your activities and pay attention to them undisturbed. Since hypnosis recordings almost always begin by inducing relaxation, they should never be listened to while you are driving or taking care of your baby, or doing anything else that requires your attention to safety. Subliminal music recordings allow much more opportunity for listening. You can listen while driving, using your computer, cleaning the house, taking a walk, or doing just about anything.

The ability to create positive internal changes by using subliminal recordings while performing rote tasks is a great benefit for a busy mom. While you're listening to the audible music, your subconscious mind is absorbing inaudible subliminal messages that create a positive effect.

CHAPTER 12

Take a Break—Relaxation and Stress Management

If you are distressed by anything external, the pain is not due to the thing itself, but to your estimate of it; and this you have the power to revoke at any moment.

~ MARCUS AURELIUS

Remember those old, "Calgon, take me away!" television commercials? They were on the right track. Sometimes you just need to lose yourself in a bubble bath. If you have a supportive partner helping you with the baby, it is entirely possible you might be able to sneak away for half an hour. Even if you're on your own or if your schedule just doesn't allow it, there are still relaxation and stress management techniques you can try.

The Effect of Stress on the Body

Postpartum depression can bring with it a host of symptoms, including anxiety and stress, and stress brings its own attendant symptoms, like insomnia.

Stress can produce a range of symptoms including headache, insomnia and high blood pressure. It can make you tired and give you an upset stomach (and even an ulcer at chronic levels). It can knot-up your muscles and leave you too anxious to make them relax. Stress can also cause hair loss, often reversible after the stress is brought under control. Stress can also cause weight gain if you're eating for emotional reasons or turning to high-calorie, high-carbohydrate comfort foods.

Cortisol, the Stress Hormone

One of the reasons stress causes physical change is that the adrenal glands release cortisol during stressful situations, such as in an emergency or when you are suddenly surprised or frightened by something. Cortisol plays an important function in the body. If there really is a life-endangering situation, cortisol gives you a burst of speed and power so you can fight or escape to safety. This is known as the "fight-or-flight" response. Cortisol is also part of the immune system, responds to inflammation, helps metabolize glucose and maintain blood sugar levels, and helps to regulate blood pressure.

In a situation where levels of stress are high for long periods of time, or in instances of chronic stress, cortisol can interfere with thought processes, suppress thyroid function, and raise blood pressure.

Fortunately, there are steps you can take at home to combat stress. The do-it-yourself aspect of stress control offers the added benefit of making you feel that you're taking steps to be in control of your own life—that alone can help start lowering stress.

Meditation

There are many different approaches to meditation, ranging from free-spirited to guided meditation. You can count breaths, repeat a specific word or phrase, stare at a candle flame or try a system like Zen meditation or transcendental meditation. In guided meditation, a guide leads you through imagery or visualization, taking you to peaceful surroundings or helping you to focus on goals. What is important with meditation is consistency—to keep doing whatever it is that feels right, centering your mind and body.

There may be many different paths to get there, but all forms of meditation share some features— usually a narrowing of focus, relaxed breathing and concentration on a specific word, thought or idea. Medical science hasn't quite been able to explain what meditation does, but studies have shown that people who practice meditation for a six- to eight-week period experience a reduction in both physical and emotional stress. According to some studies, the immune systems of meditation practitioners are activated less often and their response to stressors is lessened.

Medical science may not fully understand this mind-body connection, or why the immune system calms to meditation, but the evidence exists. There is also evidence of increased electrical activity in the left frontal lobe during meditation—electrical activity in that region of the brain is associated with optimism.

According to the website MayoClinic.com, meditation can help you learn to gain a new perspective on stressful situations, build stress management skills, increase self-awareness, focus on the present and reduce negative emotions, all of which can be beneficial to a new mother coping with postpartum depression.

If you try meditation and it doesn't come easily, cut yourself some slack. Meditation takes practice and some methods may work better for you than others. If one form doesn't work for you, another might.

Deep Breathing

When you become tense, you might find that you're taking fast, shallow breaths, the same way you would if you were to hyperventilate. Stress speeds up breathing and heart rate as the body, which thinks it's in danger, prepares to decide what it needs to do to save itself.

Deep breathing is a simple response to stress, a technique you can practice anywhere at any time. Simply concentrate on taking in your breath and feeling the air travel all the way through your body. You can control your breathing by breathing in for a slow three count, hold it for a count of three, and breathe out for twice as long—an old meditation technique that focuses your attention on your breath and off of whatever stressors were making you anxious.

Yoga

Yoga connects mind and body. Through slow, controlled movement and breathing, you concentrate on finding and maintaining poses, letting extraneous thoughts slide away and stretching out the kinks and knots in your muscles. Yoga, an ancient tradition started in India and spread worldwide, requires concentration and physical dexterity. It can distract you from repetitive, stressful or distressing thoughts and can help un-cramp and un-fold muscles held rigid because of stress.

Yoga can also help you lose weight and tone up muscles after your pregnancy. It can help you become more flexible and comfortable in your body again, which can give you back some of the self-confidence that may be missing due to postpartum depression.

If you can get to a class with a certified instructor, you'll be able to learn in a supportive environment and have someone to correct and help refine your poses. You'll also be out in the world again, socializing, which can have a salutary effect on depression and stress. Look for drop-in classes, baby-and-me classes or yoga centers that offer childcare.

If you cannot get out to a class, there are DVDs that offer instruction and there are many qualified instructors presenting free, short YouTube videos that may fit into the time you have available.

Massage

Some studies show that massage can do you as much good as antidepressants, but who needs medical research to tell you that massage feels good? Even a short neck rub can make you feel less stressed. Sometimes removing the physical manifestations of stress can help relieve the psychological feelings of stress.

The idea behind using massage as a tool to combat stress is the mind-body connection. Using massage to help heal the body from the effects of stress can help you relax and help the body feel more calm and in control. Massage releases endorphins into your system, which may make you slightly groggy as well as relaxed after a massage. Massage also triggers alpha brainwaves, which are slower, more relaxed and more creative brainwaves than beta brainwaves, which are experienced in the waking state. Massage also releases neurotransmitters in your system— serotonin, which effects mood and appetite and helps regulate sleep, and dopamine, which triggers the brain's pleasure centers and regulates emotion.

Acupuncture

Medical studies that measure physical responses to stress (heart rate, blood pressure, electrical activity of the brain) have shown that acupuncture is highly successful at relieving stress.

Acupuncture is a component of Traditional Chinese Medicine that treats ailments of body and spirit through the use of very thin needles. The practice treats the entire body and spirit holistically and is generally used in conjunction with exercise and dietary changes.

According to Western medicine, acupuncture works because it stimulates systems such as the nervous system into releasing hormones and chemicals that the body needs to function properly, such as white blood cells, thyroid hormones and endorphins (the body's natural pain-killer). According to Asian medicine, acupuncture works because it releases the body's Chi or Qi—flow of energy. The goal is to achieve balance in the energies of the body, which is achieved by inserting very thin needles (about the thickness of a single hair) into key locations on the body in order to align the energies of the elements—wood, fire, metal, water and earth.

Acupuncture is a safe stress relief option with relatively no side effects. In many cases acupuncture results in increased energy levels, and the increased flow of blood and brain stimulation can help the body and mind combat depression. A course of treatments, maybe 12 to 18 in all, can result in long-term relief.

Find What You Love

Finding pleasure in the things you love doing is one of the simplest steps you can take to reduce stress and feel better. In a depressed state, this is possibly one of the more difficult things to do. Even so, you can start with the basics: what are your favorite things to do? We all have those things we enjoy, activities that once we start, we are apt to forget the time and all the other things we were supposed to be doing. If you love to read or write or paint, or do any creative thing, giving yourself the gift of time to pursue these activities is a wonderful stress release. If you love to read mysteries or thrillers or romances or nonfiction, just curling up with a book can significantly lower your stress. Do you love to cook? Or run? Or garden? Whatever it is that gives you pleasure, indulging in the activity can help lower your stress levels.

One hurdle is convincing yourself that it's OK to take the time to do these things. For many, the stress is compounded by the feeling that you're supposed to be doing more than you are. For a new mother struggling with postpartum depression, feelings of guilt and worthlessness can make it difficult to even feel that you deserve to take steps to feel better, and depression can make it hard to feel enjoyment in activities you normally love.

You deserve to find what you love again and to use those activities to help manage stress. Talking care of yourself is essential in handling your postpartum depression, and taking care of yourself is essential if you're going to be able to take care of your baby. Finding joy in the things you love, and pursuing them as stress management tools, is no more self-indulgent than taking a multivitamin so that you can stay healthy and care for your family.

CHAPTER 13

Breathe—Herbs and Aromatherapy

*Nothing is more memorable than a smell. One scent can be
unexpected, momentary and fleeting, yet conjure up a childhood
summer beside a lake in the mountains.*

~ DIANE ACKERMAN

The sense of smell can evoke emotions in a heartbeat. Some of our strongest memories are associated with scent, and various smells transport us instantly—think of summer barbecues being lit across the neighborhood or the evergreen smell of a Christmas tree. The brain supplies nearly instant associations with these smells, and your mood can alter according to the association.

Aromatherapy is the therapeutic use of essential oils to comfort and heal by using scent to activate sensory channels in the brain. It relies on our sense of smell and the way nose and brain work together to cause changes in mood. The therapy has been used in cultures from India and Egypt to China, Greece and Rome for over 6,000 years. While U.S. medicine is slow and cautious in catching on (or at least to admitting that aromatherapy produces results), some European countries not only embrace the therapy but have made it part of their mainstream healthcare; in France, for example, some essential oils can only be prescribed by a doctor. In the U.S., however, aromatherapy remains among the category of alternate therapies.

The herbs used in aromatherapy are reduced to essential oils, which are created by concentrating extracts from the petals, blossoms, leaves, stems, seeds and/or roots of plants. The oils contain properties that make them effective in relieving physical or emotional conditions, promoting health and relaxation, or for use in antibacterial, antiviral and antifungal preparations and the like.

If you visit an aromatherapist, he or she will probably ask how you're feeling and what concerns have brought you in. The aromatherapist will also ask you about your general medical background, stressors in your life, and exercise and diet.

It's Not All About Breathing In

The way aromatherapy is thought to work doesn't rely solely on inhalation of the oils used in the practice. The term actually refers to many traditional therapies such as massage therapy when those therapies incorporate essential oils. There are several different ways that aromatherapy herbs and oils are used, including:

- Diffusion (where the oils are dispersed into the air and inhaled)

- Direct inhalation

- Topical application (during aromatherapy massage, in which essential oils are mixed with a carrier oil and massaged into the skin, or for use in bath or in skincare products)

Make sure you never apply pure essential oil directly to the skin. They must be diluted in mixtures with other oils or beauty products. Side effects can include a burn-like rash or allergic reactions. Any kind of infusion that involves taking essential oils by mouth should only be provided by a professional aromatherapist, as ingestion can be toxic.

Why It Works

The theory behind aromatherapy is that the inhalation of the herbal scent stimulates the limbic system—structures in the brain that include the amygdale and hippocampus, which control emotions and store memories.

When used in conjunction with massage as topical oils, essential oils can activate thermal receptors, and, as some evidence suggests, they are absorbed through the skin and can be measured by blood test within five to twenty minutes. Aromatherapy massage with essential oils is thought to relieve depression, possibly because the oils stimulate positive emotions and stimulate the memory center of the brain.

Depending on the herbs used, the desired effect may be to feel more relaxed and calm, to encourage sleep, or to feel wide awake and stimulated. In one study, sixteen new mothers were given aromatherapy massage during the first two days after giving birth and showed significantly fewer postpartum-depression symptoms than the control group who did not receive massage.

Relieving Symptoms

Essential oils can be used in aromatherapy for a variety of reasons. For physical ailments, benefits can include relief from

- Body and muscular aches
- Headaches
- Circulatory problems
- Stomach upset
- Menstrual concerns

- Menopause problems
- Insomnia

In the emotional realm, aromatherapy can have a beneficial effect on

- Anxiety
- Stress
- Depression

Especially important to a new mother is the connection between aromatherapy and sleep. By triggering the limbic system with a soothing scent, the brain itself will work to relax the various parts of the body holding tension and even cause the body to become sleepy.

The Oils

The following is a list of some of the more popular essential oils used in aromatherapy:

Aniseed: contains estrogen-like compounds that may help with PMS and menopausal symptoms.

Basil: good for concentration and mental clarity; can help with depression; used to treat headaches.

Bergamot: a sleep balm, good for treating depression, promotes digestive and urinary tract health; used with eucalyptus it's good for the skin.

Chamomile: frequently brewed as a tea, promotes relaxation and a feeling of wellbeing.

Clove oil: a topical painkiller; antispasmodic; prevents nausea and vomiting.

Fennel: contains estrogen-like compounds that may help with PMS and menopausal symptoms.

Jasmine: used as an aphrodisiac.

Lavender oil: antiseptic; headache relief; can aid in insomnia relief, calms the nerves, deepens sleep.

Lemon oil: lifts mood; relieves stress; relieves depression.

Mandarin: has a balancing and calming effect; used for insomnia.

Naroli: a natural sedative, it can help relieve anxiety and insomnia.

Orange oil: this citrus oil can relieve depression and lift mood; can increase concentration.

Rose oil: used to relieve anxiety, stress and depression.

Sage and clary sage: contains estrogen-like compounds that may help with PMS and menopausal symptoms; clary sage can make you drowsy.

Sandalwood: sometimes considered an aphrodisiac; relieves stress; relieves depression; has a calming effect.

Thyme oil: for relief from nervousness, stress and fatigue.

Ylang Ylang: sometimes considered an aphrodisiac; relieves stress and anger, promotes relaxation.

Aromatherapy Products

For the do-it-yourself-at-home version of aromatherapy, there are a variety of products on the market. You can find soothing, stress-relieving herbs in neck wraps, sleep pillows and eye pillows, and many of those can be heated or chilled to provide extra relief. Aromatherapy bath oils and bath salts turn your bath into a healing experience. Aromatherapy candles can scent the air and create a healing environment. You can also find diffusers or burners that heat essential oils slowly, releasing the scent into the air.

When looking at products to use at home, look for those that use actual essential oils rather than those simply designed to smell like the herb.

Aromatherapy uses a holistic approach to treat physical and emotional disorders, or simply to promote relaxation and sound sleep. The products are natural and largely side-effect free, but there are a few things to keep in mind. First of all, read labels. Many of the aromatherapy massage oils consist of natural scent added to a neutral oil, which can be a nut oil and thus a problem for anyone with an allergy to nuts. People with asthma or allergies, skin conditions or high blood pressure, or who have epilepsy or have ever had a seizure, should take care when working with aromatherapy. Remember also that essential oils are flammable, so keep them away from open flames. Women who are breastfeeding or pregnant should check with their doctor before starting an aromatherapy regimen.

Just stopping to take stock of your life and taking a deep breath can sometimes make you feel better when you're struggling with postpartum depression. Add aromatherapy essential oils to that mix and you may find your mood improving even faster.

CHAPTER 14

Speak Up—The Power of Therapy

My definition of success is total self acceptance. We can obtain all of the material possessions we desire quite easily; however, attempting to change our deepest thoughts and learning to love ourselves is a monumental challenge.

~ FRANKI

Traditional western medicine treats the body more than the mind. Holistic and natural approaches, often known as alternative medicine in the West, treat the whole person—body, mind and emotion.

Therapy, also known as psychotherapy and talk therapy, can take the body into account but mostly focuses on the mind and the emotions. For a new mother experiencing the symptoms of postpartum depression, talking with a therapist can provide an outlet for confusing or overwhelming thoughts and emotions, as well as help to create plans for solutions.

Therapy can help you find a healthy outlet for your emotions and develop healthy problem-solving techniques and coping skills. By talking with a psychiatrist, psychologist or certified counselor, you can discuss what you want to accomplish, find books and online sources that provide guidance and support, and learn how to set realistic, achievable goals.

Some of the conditions where therapy can help include anxiety and mood disorders, stress, and depression. In addition, therapy can help you transition through major life changes and work on sleeping better.

Talk Therapy

Talk therapy is a simple, natural and powerful tool for a woman struggling with postpartum depression. Together, therapist and new mother can work through different therapeutic approaches, including cognitive-behavioral, interpersonal and family therapy.

Talk therapy offers you a time and place to express all those confusing emotions and stressors in an environment where you are provided positive guidance and support. A therapist can also offer a structured pace and method for moving forward—in place of jumbled thoughts and feelings, a trained therapist can help you sort out what you're feeling and prioritize the most important aspects to deal with first.

Cognitive Behavioral Therapy

This type of therapy focuses on making actual changes to behavior and increasing self-awareness. By talking with a therapist in regular sessions, you learn to focus on thoughts, emotions and behaviors that are not serving you and are negative, repetitive or unwanted. By learning to recognize when you are falling into thought or behavioral patterns that are negative, you can learn to control and regulate your thoughts and actions, even if the situation around you has not changed. This type of therapy may incorporate journaling or keeping an emotions diary or chart that helps you identify times of day and situations that may be causing or exacerbating the negative emotions. Likewise, charting can help you identify the times and situations that encourage positive emotions.

Cognitive behavioral therapy can help make you feel more in control of your thoughts, emotions and life and can teach you coping skills that will continue to help you even after your recovery from postpartum depression.

This type of therapy allows you to discuss with the therapist the stresses in your life and identify those that are giving you the most problems. Then you can work with the therapist to put together an action plan, setting realistic and workable goals for improving those areas of your life. Sometimes just having a plan of action can make you feel more in control of a chaotic situation. This type of therapy can also help you transition into new routines in your life while staying true to who you are. Many new mothers feel stressed by the idea that they have taken on a new identity and are no longer the same person after giving birth. If this sounds like you, this type of therapy can help you piece together your identity and move into the future more confidently.

Interpersonal Therapy

Interpersonal therapy can be especially helpful for you as a new mother as you try to get a routine together and make sense of all the changes in your life with the addition of the baby. It is another form of talk therapy that focuses on interpersonal relationships and helps you develop better interpersonal communication skills.

Family Therapy

Family therapy can help everyone in the family come together to deal with the stresses of the new baby and new routines.

Group Therapy and Support Groups

Group therapy involves a small group of people coming together to share similar concerns in a group led by a therapist. Interaction with people facing similar new challenges can be comforting and inspirational.

Support groups are a great option for new mothers who are feeling isolated and alone in their depression. Sometimes just knowing that other people are going through the same things as you and are looking for and finding their own solutions can help.

Support groups give you a chance to talk with other new mothers who are feeling insecure about new body issues or parenting styles or are coping with depression at a time when they expected to be feeling joy. There are support groups for mothers and support groups for couples, where you and your partner can both receive positive guidance. Support groups can also be a great place to meet new friends.

Therapy Tools

Your therapist will have a variety of tools he or she works with frequently, some of which may involve emotion or depression diaries or plan sheets that allow you to track your emotions. Some are as simple as a grid for each week where you fill out how you feel at various times of day and rate your depression on a scale (likely a 1 to 10 scale). If you fill out the diary on a regular basis, you and your therapist will be able to see patterns emerge. You may find that certain times of day, situations or interactions have a positive or negative effect on your mood. This information can help you make changes to improve your mood and monitor and control your emotions.

How to Find a Therapist Who's Right for You

So how do you find the right therapist for you? One way is to ask your doctor for a referral. Another is to check with the psychological association for your state (the state's psychological association website may have quite a bit of information on therapy and various mood disorders that you may find useful as well).

If you have health insurance through an employer, you should be able to find a referral through your plan. In addition, if you are comfortable seeking help through your employer, some employee assistance programs offer counseling services or referrals.

Before your first appointment, make a list of what you want to discuss with the therapist. The first meeting will probably be spent getting to know each other so the therapist can understand what issues you're facing and what outcomes you would like to reach. It may take several meetings for you and the therapist to decide how best to approach the issues and concerns with which you're seeking help.

The first meeting is also your chance to ask questions of the therapist, to find out what his or her approach to therapy is, and how he or she plans to work with you. Some of your questions for the therapist may include what type of therapy you'll be undergoing and what outcomes the therapist feels are possible.

If you are not comfortable with the therapist, look for another referral to someone else. You need to be comfortable with the therapist so that you can concentrate on the concerns that brought you to therapy.

Organizations That Can Help You Locate a Therapist

National Alliance on Mental Illness (NAMI)
www.nami.org
Lists resources by state and community. Should be able to provide referrals.

Mental Health America
http://www.mentalhealthamerica.net/
Extensive lists by state and therapy upon clicking the red "Get Help" button.

Confidentiality

If you decide to seek help via talk therapy, you should know that your conversations with your therapist are completely confidential under law, except in a few rare situations (for example, if a patient is threatening to hurt herself or someone in her care, the therapist would be required by law to report to law enforcement). You can talk about anything, and because the relationship is limited to therapy and the therapist is outside your "normal life," it is a chance to work towards understanding your emotions, fears, frustrations and challenges in a safe, supportive, creative and goal-oriented space. The more honest you can be with your therapist, the more you will be able to get out of therapy.

It can take time to see results from therapy, but during that time, the support from your therapist can make life more manageable.

CHAPTER 15

Brighten Up Your Life— Light Therapy

Keep your face to the sun and you will never see the shadows.

~ HELEN KELLER

L ight therapy (also known as bright light therapy and phototherapy) was developed to treat people suffering from Seasonal Affective Disorder, or SAD. SAD is a type of mood disorder that commonly occurs in fall and winter months when the days are shorter and there is less direct sunlight or natural light. Sunlight triggers the neurotransmitters in the brain, stimulating the brain's production of serotonin. Lowered levels of serotonin lead to depression.

SAD and PPD share a variety of symptoms, as they are both mood disorders involving depression. Symptoms they have in common include depression itself, impulse eating, lack of energy, fatigue, trouble concentrating, lowered desire to spend time with friends and family, and sometimes hypersomnia (sleeping excessively). Postpartum depression can add anxiety, insomnia, low self-esteem, feelings of worthlessness and guilt into the mix.

Medical science is studying the effects of light therapy, with encouraging results, on people diagnosed with SAD and on people suffering from other types of depression, obsessive-compulsive disorders and sleep disturbances—all of which can occur with postpartum depression.

Could You Have Both PPD and SAD?

SAD-like symptoms do not only occur with the onset of fall and winter. People can experience SAD when they live in climates that are frequently cloudy, rainy or dark, or when they receive limited natural light because they work night shifts.

For a mother who may be staying up all night with her new baby, SAD is a risk. In addition, studies have shown that women who give birth during fall or winter are more likely to experience SAD even if they do not experience postpartum depression. Even if you have never experienced SAD before, there is a possibility that—because your hormones are already undergoing drastic changes, rising sharply during pregnancy and dropping significantly at birth—you may be more sensitive to brain chemistry changes resulting from lowered levels of natural light and therefore more apt to experience SAD. The contrary is true as well; women who experience SAD during the last trimester of pregnancy are more likely to develop PPD.

How Light Therapy Works

Light therapy is all about triggering the neurotransmitters that elevate mood. The simplest form of light therapy is just going outside and being in the natural sunlight. Even 15 minutes a day can make a difference in your mood. If you take a walk during that time, the exercise can help trigger endorphins, the body's feel-good chemical. You may even feel better about yourself for getting in the day's exercise. That's a win from all angles.

For environments with limited natural light, there is the simulated option. This involves sitting near a light box that mimics natural sunlight and filters most of the UV rays. The bright light from the light box stimulates the brain and influences it to produce more serotonin, which in turn eases depression and improves mood. It is advantageous to start the day with a light therapy session. Some light boxes can even be programmed to wake you with a dawn-like light that continues to grow in intensity until you wake up.

You can wake to your light box, work with it on your desk, or have it activated while watching television. To be effective, the light needs to enter your eyes, so sleeping through the light therapy sessions would not be effective. Most sessions start in quarter hour chunks of time, gradually increasing up to two hours. Light therapy is better used in the morning, as using it at night can interrupt sleep patterns.

Light therapy is considered safe, and side effects are rare and usually mild. If you do experience side effects, they should not last long. Bright light therapy can cause mania in rare cases, much the same way the non-setting summer sun in Alaska can cause a bipolar-like mania and prevent people from sleeping.

If you are using light therapy in part because PPD is causing sleep disturbances, you should be aware that sleep disturbances can be a side effect to the therapy, along with headaches and eyestrain. None of the side effects are particularly serious and will, at any rate, pass after a week or two. As long as your eyes are not overly sensitive to light, light therapy may offer you a simple, natural solution to postpartum depression and sleep disturbances.

The effectiveness of light therapy can be enhanced by choosing the right light box. Different intensities and lengths of treatment have been studied. Results show that lights producing 10,000 lux (which is the measure of intensity of light as perceived by the human eye) and used for 30 minutes are the most effective. Since morning light has been shown to be very beneficial in beating depression, some lights will simulate dawn over a period of a quarter hour up to an hour and a half. (You can set the time to suit your preference.) The simulated dawn provides a gentle wakening as well as the first light therapy session of the day.

Consistency is another key to success. Do not skip phototherapy sessions and do try to use the light box around the same time every day.

If light therapy works for you, it will probably be by lessening depression symptoms—not by curing the PPD. But if you start to have more energy and are better-rested and happier, you will be in a better position to manage your postpartum depression.

CHAPTER 16:

Take Notes—The Art of Journaling

We write to taste life twice, in the moment and in retrospect.
~ ANAÏS NIN

Getting your thoughts on paper can be tremendously freeing and very helpful as you move through your postpartum depression. A journal is one place you can be absolutely honest about every emotion—the positive, the negative and the confusing.

Journaling can be considered a form of self-therapy. You are giving yourself permission to open up about everything that is bothering you (and everything that's making you happy—you don't have to limit yourself to anything!) When journaling in a time of crisis or depression, you will be writing in what is often called a depression journal or a mood journal, but opening it up to everything that's going on for you can make it a life journal.

In your own journal you are free to record whatever you are feeling without fear of being judged. Sometimes in addition to dealing with confusing or upsetting emotions as a new mother struggling with PPD, you might also harbor the fear of being judged unfit. Postpartum depression symptoms include anxiety, uncertainty, feelings of guilt and worthlessness—adding on the fear that people will judge you and declare you an unfit mother can make the stress even worse.

Putting down your thoughts and feelings on paper can help you understand them. Whether you are dealing with fear, anxiety, stress, depression, exhaustion, or relationship concerns, all of it can come out on paper in a personal, private space.

Records and Rewards

Some of the benefits of journaling include having a written record that can show you at a glance your progress through depression. If you have written in a journal consistently during your struggles with your postpartum mood disorder, glancing back over previous entries can prove to you how far you've come. Journaling can also give you a written record of how you've dealt with (and triumphed over) adversity in the past. If you experienced postpartum depression after previous pregnancies, a long-time journal is a reminder that the mood disorder is temporary—you have gone through it before and triumphed. You can do it again.

You may also find that by simply opening the floodgates and letting everything out on paper, you discover that what you thought was bothering you is not actually the main stressor or depressor. Conversely, you may find that something you thought was a minor stress is actually significant. Problems you viewed as major stumbling blocks may now appear to have an easy solution.

You can use a journal to brainstorm solutions to problems, to try and understand complex, confusing emotions, or just to vent. Sometimes if a depression hangs on, it is easy to start feeling that you're going to alienate the people you most need in your life, those people you can talk to about whatever is bothering you. If you're worried that you're asking too much of your support system, a journal can be the place you sift through all your concerns and select those you most want to talk to friends and family about.

Getting Started

Keeping a journal should not be a chore, and it will prove advantageous if you keep up with it regularly. Writing consistently in your journal will make it a natural part of your life, perhaps even a quiet time you look forward to.

The journal is not a place to worry about neatness. No matter what type of journal you keep, it's yours to fill in any way you choose. Neatness does not count, at least not here. You don't have to worry about grammar or spelling, penmanship or typing. No need to worry about complete sentences or whether or not you're being clear; you're the only reader (unless you choose otherwise) and you only need to be clear to yourself.

If you sit down with a notebook or a blank document on your screen and you feel a sense of panic at the blank page, don't worry. Just start writing (or typing) anything that comes to mind. The important part is to get started. There is no set amount you have to write, no quota, and there are many ways to begin. Here are some ideas for getting started:

- Pick an event or emotion that's bothering you. Write it at the top of the page and write whatever follows naturally.

- Write down a word that sums up a concern you have—it might be body or money or relationship. Then follow with whatever comes naturally and you will find your thoughts and feelings start to flow.

- Did you ever do a clustering brainstorming exercise in school? Write a word from your thoughts and feelings in the middle of the page and circle it. Then add related words to connect to it and connect more words to those words, going farther and farther out until you have a diagram of the thoughts and feelings that are bothering you. You might be surprised by the directions you take. Words that have more circles connected to them may not be the ones you expected.

- Try freewriting. Initially presented in *Writing Down the Bones* by Natalie Goldberg, free writing is a process for defeating the blank page. Take a word or sentence or title and write for a set period of time without stopping. Set a timer and write for three or five or ten minutes, paying no attention to grammar or spelling and not letting the editor in your head interrupt. Just write. Don't pause, don't think; don't let the pen (or keyboard) stop moving. The exercise can surprise you with insights, found poetry, tiny short stories, lists of concerns, lists of joys, or just five minutes' worth of looking for solutions.

There are no hard and fast rules to keeping a journal. It's whatever feels right to you. If choosing a notebook with room to paste pictures seems right, do that. If you want an ultra-neat bound journal in which you write with a special pen, that works too. The trick to journaling is simply to let yourself do it.

Types of Journals

Pen and Paper

A journal can be whatever you want it to be. You can repurpose a notebook you used in school or invest in a leather-bound, ornately designed journal. There are diary systems that allow you to add pages and keep a perpetual record, so that every July 1 follows the previous July 1, giving you a record of every July 1 (or any other day) for the past years that you've kept a journal.

Online Journals

Today's journal keepers have a variety of choices. If you are worried about privacy with a hardcopy journal, you can choose from several online systems that allow you to password protect your electronic journal. These are a great choice if you type faster than you can write by hand, and if you have online access via smartphone or tablet, you can update whenever and wherever you happen to be.

Penzu (http://penzu.com) offers free locked private journal sites or pro membership fee-paid encrypted sites for keeping your journal. Pro membership allows you to update from mobile devices and both allow you to add photos to your journal. If eventually you choose to go public with your journal, there is a sharing feature.

My Therapy Journal (www.mytherapyjournal.com) is a monthly fee site that offers not only a locked, private journal account, but also software to create charts to track your progress.

Blogs

Blogs (originally a "weblog") can be locked so that only specific friends and family can read what you have written. You can protect either individual posts or the blog in its entirety. However, if you are socially inclined, the blogosphere can introduce you to a number of other people who blog about concerns that may be similar to yours. You can use tags on your entries to sort by topic, and if you're consistent in maintaining your blog and want to make it public, you can list your blog in a variety of blog directories.

One benefit to blogging is the chance to become part of an online community of people who have similar interests (or issues) to yours. There are blogs on just about every topic in the world, some of them offering complete and well-researched material that could possibly guide you to solutions for your PPD that you otherwise might not have found.

The potential drawbacks of a blog community are directly related to the benefits. No one polices blogs, so there is no way to know if the information you're reading is accurate. Some could be well researched and others purely speculative—you just have to verify the information yourself. In addition, a community can bring with it people whose intentions are not positive and who want to share hurtful things.

If you do want to blog and make your journal public, you have an opportunity to help others who may be going through experiences and feelings similar to your own and who may be relieved to read your story—just as you may find relief reading the blogs of others dealing with concerns similar to yours.

Another choice to consider with a blog is to turn off the comments function. If you're concerned about receiving unhelpful, unsolicited and possibly hurtful comments from strangers, you can remove the option for readers to leave comments before anyone ever does.

At the time of this writing, two of the most popular blog platforms are WordPress (available at http://wordpress.com) and Blogger (accessed through Google), both of which are free at the basic level (you can upgrade and add various functionalities for a price). Both are fairly user-friendly and simple to set up. If you want your blog to be easily discovered and read, you can choose a blog host, which will help get your blog attention for a minimal monthly or annual fee, but you can also choose a completely free blog simply by signing up and letting readers find you however they can. After a certain number of posts, you can apply to be listed in free blog directories, but you have to first prove that you are a consistent blogger.

Journaling can free you up to express your emotions and enable you to create a record of where you've been and where you're going. Letting your emotions spill out without having to worry about hurting anyone's feelings or not making sense can be tremendously freeing. You can get started for free, whether you are working in a repurposed notebook or on a blog site. Journaling can be a positive step forward in your struggle against postpartum depression.

CHAPTER 17:

Rest Up—A Guide for Sleep

The best cure for insomnia is to get a lot of sleep.
~ W. C. FIELDS

S ome new mothers sleep fitfully. Others don't sleep at all. And almost no one with a new baby in the household gets the full, prescribed eight hours of slumber. Studies show that somewhere around 80 percent of women diagnosed with postpartum depression suffer from insomnia and sleep deprivation.

Some new mothers don't get enough sleep because they are too anxious about the new baby to fall asleep or stay asleep. They are afraid they'll miss the cry of the infant that should have awakened them, or they constantly wake, afraid something is wrong. Other women fall asleep only to wake long before they should, from nightmares or from anxiety, and find they can't fall back asleep.

Others, facing interrupted sleep because of the baby's sleep/wake cycle, find it impossible to get deep, restful sleep during the periods of time they can sleep. If you are constantly expecting to be awakened, you will likely start waking on your own, or your sleep might be shallow and not refreshing.

Lack of routine can also disrupt sleep patterns. Not all babies sleep the same number of hours every night or during the same timeframes. An unpredictable sleep schedule means the body doesn't know when it's going to get sleep again, which leads to stressful, un-refreshing sleep.

Insomnia, interrupted sleep, and sleep deprivation can all signal the onset of postpartum depression and postpartum depression in turn can cause insomnia. In fact, inability to sleep is often listed as one of the most frustrating and upsetting symptoms of postpartum depression. Some new mothers end up feeling dread at the prospect of even trying to fall asleep. It can make you feel panicky to know that you are not going to be able to get the healing, restful sleep you need before you have to get out of bed and face another stressful day.

Sleep deprivation can wreak havoc with emotions that may already be out of control. Some of the effects of sleep deprivation include:

- Anxiety
- Depression
- Physical weakness

- Difficulty concentrating
- Lack of mental clarity
- Irritability

These symptoms from sleep deprivation can exacerbate postpartum depression, or may well be symptoms of the mood disorder.

The Benefits of Sleep

Sleep serves a critical role in our health and well-being and is important for mental clarity, concentration, and emotional stability. Sleep is the time when the brain consolidates and stores memories and the body repairs itself and releases growth hormone. Many important bodily functions are impacted by inadequate sleep. Insufficient sleep has been correlated with depression, anxiety, and mental distress. Lack of sufficient sleep has also been linked to weight gain. Studies have shown that those people who are consistently sleep-deprived eat 22 percent more calories on a daily basis— approximately 550 more calories daily—which can add up to over 50 unwanted pounds in a year.

Conversely, getting enough sleep can aid weight loss. Medical research believes this to be caused by the appetite-suppressing hormone leptin, which body fat releases during sleep. Leptin can help you lose weight in your sleep, but you have to be able to sleep in order to activate it.

Find the Time to Sleep

Hoping to get eight hours of uninterrupted sleep while you're caring for your newborn may be too optimistic. Infants may fall asleep six to eight times during a 24-hour period and spend as much as 16 to 18 hours sleeping. However, during that stretch of time they are apt to wake every two to four hours with needs that must be met.

Studies have shown that if you can get a four-hour stretch of time to sleep without interruption, in addition to catching some shorter periods of sleep during the day, you will feel better and function better. Trade off with your partner if you can, taking turns caring for your baby at night, so that both of you can have at least a four-hour stretch of sleep.

You may also find that it helps to keep the baby closer to you when you're sleeping. If you don't have to go as far to respond to your baby at night, you may be able to fall back to sleep more quickly.

Getting enough sleep may be difficult. At times, even attempting to do so may seem counterproductive, as simply trying to get to sleep may feel stressful. Changing your sleeping patterns is never easy, as anyone who has ever worked a graveyard shift can attest; humans are diurnal—

awake during the day, asleep at night. Making a change and dealing with shorter sleep cycles is hard. In order to get adequate rest, many experts suggest that you sleep when your baby sleeps. If that doesn't work, ask your partner or another trusted friend or family member to watch your baby for short periods of time so you can nap. Ask for help—you don't have to be super woman right now.

Natural Sleep Solutions

New research shows that treating insomnia can often help treat depression. Fortunately, there are many natural sleep solutions you can use to help get that deep, restful sleep you so desire. Here are some steps you can take to assist with sleep:

- Engage in calming and relaxing exercise, like yoga or deep stretching.

- De-stress as best you can before turning in. Refrain from doing anything stimulating or stressful for at least 30 minutes before bed. The body releases cortisol when you're stressed, which is not conducive to sleep.

- Try watching something mindless on television or read a book you enjoy. Avoid dramas and thrillers.

- Take a warm bath. Raising your body temperature can help you sleep, and the warmth will relax knotted muscles.

- Use some aromatherapy bath salts or bath oils during your warm bath to encourage sleep.

- Listen to soothing music.

- Write in your journal. To calm a worried or overactive mind, write your thoughts and concerns in your journal. Writing it down allows you to release it from your head onto the paper, freeing your mind of concerns when you turn out the lights.

- Use your bed for sleep and intimacy only—no discussions about finances, no watching TV— just a peaceful place to sleep.

- Create a restful environment in your bedroom—dark, quiet, and uncluttered.

- Expose yourself to at least 20 minutes of natural daylight (or light therapy) every day. Sunlight triggers specific chemicals like melatonin which are beneficial to getting restful sleep.

- Listen to a hypnosis recording for sleep.

In addition to the suggestions above, try to maintain a regular routine. Go to bed at the same time and get up at the same time, or as close as possible. The body adapts to routine and will adapt to a routine that does not promote sleep if you let it.

A routine can help your baby sleep better, too, and the better your baby sleeps, the better you can sleep. Try creating a stimulating environment between your baby's naps, to keep him or her awake and engaged. When your baby naps during the day, don't block out light or lower sounds, and instead continue life as usual. When your baby sleeps at night, encourage that sleep by keeping the room dim or dark and quiet. You can also help your baby adjust to a pattern by performing routine actions at night—a bath for the baby, clean clothes, a set bedtime.

Some things to avoid before bedtime:

- Caffeine

- Eating simple carbohydrates (refined sugar and flour) because of the energy rush you'll get from them (see *Chapter 7: Healthy Diet— You're Still Eating for Two*)

- Eating within two to three hours of going to bed

- Vigorous exercise right before bed

- Alcohol—it may make you sleepy at first, but it interrupts sleep cycles and is a depressant

Some things you may want to initially avoid because they interfere with sleep:

- Antihistamines and decongestants

- Sedatives

- Appetite suppressants and diet pills

Some foods that may help you sleep are fresh fruits, legumes, hazel nuts, various seeds, and foods that contain tryptophan, like dairy products, turkey and mashed potatoes (think: Thanksgiving food coma).

Exercise

Studies show that exercise extends sleep duration and deepens sleep into a more restful experience. The more fit you are, the deeper your sleep and the slower your resting brain waves. But you don't have to be marathon-fit to get the benefit. Any daytime exercise, performed preferably in the morning, can help fatigue the body as well as release endorphins (natural painkillers, or feel-good hormones) and burn cortisol (the anxiety and stress hormone) all of which can make you sleep, and sleep better. The exercise/sleep connection works better if you exercise early in the day, so as not to excite the body before bedtime.

Aromatherapy for Sleep

Aromatherapy uses essential oils in massage oils, as bath oils or salts, and as inhalants from a candle or diffuser. For sleep and relaxation purposes, you can also use herb-stuffed sleep pillows, eye pillows and neck wraps, many of which can either be heated in the microwave or chilled in the freezer to provide additional comfort and healing.

Connections between the brain and the nose allow scent organs to transfer what you inhale and trigger responses in the brain. See *Chapter 13: Breathe— Herbs and Aromatherapy*, for more information on the topic.

While there is a more thorough discussion of herbs and their uses in Chapter 13, here are some of the top herbs for helping you feel relaxed or sleepy and for promoting a good night's sleep:

- Lavender: calms the nerves, muscle relaxant

- Chamomile: calming effect, relaxes mind and body

- Bergamot: sleep balm, often used with other essential oils to treat depression and anxiety

- Clary sage: has a relaxing effect, soothing and calming

- Neroli oil: natural sedative when inhaled that can help relieve anxiety; essential for people suffering from insomnia

- Sandalwood: has a potent calming effect on the nerves and digestive system; its woody scent is often used as an aid to meditation

- Ylang-Ylang: sweet, invigorating scent said to be an aphrodisiac; known for its relaxing effect on the nervous system, this herb is frequently used to treat stress and anger

- Mandarin: has a balancing, calming effect; used for insomnia

A Sleep log is included in the appendix of this book to help you keep track of important factors that can influence your sleep. The log will help you keep track of the actions you take every day and how they may be affecting your sleep.

CHAPTER 18:

Putting It All Together

Nobody can go back and start a new beginning, but anyone can start today and make a new ending.

~ MARIA ROBINSON

Congratulations! You are on your way to feeling good again using natural, healthy therapies.

The natural approaches you have read about in this book to improve your physical and emotional health during the postpartum period are quite simple. You have learned how the mind-body connection works, and you have learned about various natural treatment options including exercise, healthy diet, hypnosis, relaxation, and light therapy, to name a few.

Though this information may not seem earth shatteringly new, as a new mom suffering with postpartum depression, you may not have known how truly effective each of these natural remedies can be. Or perhaps you have felt so overwhelmed, exhausted, or stressed, you didn't know where or how to start implementing them into your daily life—just when you needed them most. The good news is that you have taken a very important first step by reading this book. But it shouldn't end there. I encourage you to take the time and effort to use the natural therapies in this book. You can use them on your own, or with the additional help of the *Creating Postpartum Wellness Program Guide*. You can obtain the program guide by going to the Postpartum Living website at www.postpartum-living.com/program. The guide offers an easy-to-follow six-week program, with step-by-step action plans for success. Also included in the Program Guide:

- Easy-to-print version of the Edinburg Postpartum Test to take to your doctor

- Six full page copies of a detailed Daily Mood Chart to track your actions and moods for the six week program

- Six full page copies of the Sleep Log to record how you are sleeping and what may be affecting your sleep for six weeks

- Six full page copies of the Physical Activity Log to record your exercise for six weeks

- Shortcuts to implementing your healthy lifestyle

- Expanded nutrition and product information

- Aromatherapy recipes you can make at home

You can find many other valuable resources and tools to support your postpartum wellness at the Postpartum Living website, including professional, customized hypnosis and subliminal recordings, a forum to ask your questions or share your experiences, and updated articles and information on postpartum depression.

Appendix: Logs and Charts

The Edinburgh Postnatal Depression Scale*

Instructions: To correctly take this postpartum depression test, please select the answer which comes closest to how you have felt during the past seven days only—not just how you feel today.

Answer the following ten questions by choosing the appropriate response. You can take the completed test to your doctor for evaluation.

During the Past 7 Days:

1. I have been able to laugh and see the funny side of things.

    a. As much as I always could

    b. Not quite so much now

    c. Definitely not so much now

    d. Not at all

2. I have looked forward with enjoyment to things.

    a. As much as I ever did

    b. Rather less than I used to

    c. Definitely less than I used to

    d. Hardly at all

3. I have blamed myself unnecessarily when things went wrong.

    a. Yes, most of the time

    b. Yes, some of the time

    c. Not very often

    d. No, never

4. I have been anxious or worried for no good reason.

    a. No, not at all

    b. Hardly ever

    c. Yes, sometimes

    d. Yes, very often

5. I have felt scared or panicky for no good reason.

    a. Yes, quite a lot

    b. Yes, sometimes

    c. No, not much

    d. No, not at all

6. Things have been getting on top of me.

    a. Yes, most of the time I haven't been able to cope at all

    b. Yes, sometimes I haven't been coping as well as usual

    c. No, most of the time I have coped quite well

    d. No, I have been coping as well as ever

7. I have been so unhappy that I have had difficulty sleeping.

   a. Yes, most of the time

   b. Yes, some of the time

   c. Not very often

   d. No, not at all

8. I have felt sad or miserable.

   a. Yes, most of the time

   b. Yes, some of the time

   c. Not very often

   d. No, not at all

9. I have been so unhappy that I have been crying.

   a. Yes, most of the time

   b. Yes, quite often

   c. Only occasionally

   d. No, never

10. The thought of harming myself has occurred to me.

    a. Yes, quite often

    b. Sometimes

    c. Hardly ever

    d. Never

*Source: J.L. Cox, J.M. Holden, and R. Sagovsky, "Detection of Postnatal Depression: Development of the 10-item Edinburgh Postnatal Depression Scale," *British Journal of Psychiatry* 150 (1987): 782-86.

Physical Activity Log

Physical Activity Log

Make a copy of this Physical Activity Log to keep track of your exercise for each week. Include the type of activity, amount of time in minutes, as well as intensity.

Week Of _____

Day of week	Type Of Activity (walked with baby, yoga, etc.)	Amount Of Time (in minutes)	Intensity (low, moderate, high)
Monday			
Tuesday			
Wednesday			
Thursday			
Friday			
Saturday			
Sunday			

Sleep Log

Sleep Log

Your sleep log will help you keep track of important factors that may be affecting your sleep. Using this log, you will be able to easily view the actions you have taken every day and how they may be affecting your sleep.

Week of: _____

Day Of The Week	SUN	MON	TUES	WED	THUR	FRI	SAT
Did you take a nap during the day?							
Did you listen to a sleep hypnosis recording?							
Did you practice relaxation or stress relief?							
Did you exercise?							
Did you get exposure to sunlight or light box?							
Did you eat at least 3 hours before bed?							
Did you take a sleep aid or herbal sleep aid?							
How much caffeine did you have?							
How much alcohol did you have?							
Other possible factors (ie: took cold medicine, baby was sick, etc.)							
Rate Quality Of Sleep From 1 – 10 (10 = Excellent/slept like a baby) (1 = Poor/wide awake or tossed and turned)							

Resources

To support your continued exploration into the natural therapies included in this book, provided is a list of resources for help, information, and support, including alternative healthcare organizations and associations as well as a list of recommended readings.

Creating Postpartum Wellness Program Resources

Supplemental program guide, audio recordings and additional resources and tools in support of the program.

Postpartum Living
www.postpartum-living.com/program

Alternative Healthcare Organizations and Associations

American Academy of Medical Acupuncture
Phone:310-364-0193
http://medicalacupuncture.org

American Association of Drugless Practitioners
Phone:903-843-6401
www.aadp.net

American Association of Naturopathic Physicians
Phone:206-298-0126
www.naturopathic.org

American Herbalists Guild
Phone:770-751-6021
www.americanherbalistsguild.com

American Holistic Health Association
Phone: 714-779-6152
www.ahha.org

American Holistic Medical Association
Phone: 703-556-9245
www.holisticmedicine.org

American Holistic Nurses Association
Phone: 800-278-2462
www.ahna.org

American Naturopathic Medical Association
Phone: 702-897-7053
http://anma.net

Associated Bodywork and Massage Professionals
Phone: 303-674-0859
www.abmp.com

Complementary Medical Association
Phone: 0845 129 8434
www.the-cma.org.uk

Doulas of North America
Phone: 888-788-3662
www.dona.org

Holistic Pediatric Association
Phone: 707-237-5312
www.hpakids.org

International Chiropractic Pediatric Association
Phone: 610-565-2360
www.icpa4kids.com

National Acupuncture Detoxification Association
Phone: 888-765-NADA
http:// www.acudetox.com/

National Center for Complementary and Alternative Medicine
Phone: 888-644-6226
http://nccam.nih.gov

National Center for Homeopathy
Phone: 703-548-7790
http://www.homeopathic.org

The National Institute of Ayurvedic Medicine
Phone: 888-246-NIAM
www.niam.com

North American Society of Homeopaths (NASH)
Phone: 206-720-7000
www.homeopathy.org

National Association of Holistic Aromatherapy
Phone: 919-917-7491
www.naha.org

Recommended Reading

Meditation and Mindfulness:
Santorelli, S. *Heal Thy Self: Lessons on Mindfulness in Medicine*. New York: Bell Tower, 2000.

Kabat-Zinn, J. *Letting Everything Become Your Teacher: 100 Lessons in Mindfulness*. New York: Delta Trade Paperbacks, 2009.

Kabat-Zinn, J. *Full Catastrophe Living: Using the Wisdom of Your Body and Mind to Face Stress, Pain and Illness*. New York: Delta Trade Paperbacks, 1991.

Aromatherapy:
Keville, K. *Aromatherapy: A Complete Guide to the Healing Art*. New York: Crossing Press, 2009.

Woorwood, V. *The Complete Book of Essential Oils and Aromatherapy: Over 600 Natural, Non-Toxic and Fragrant Recipes to Create Health– Beauty – a Safe Home Environment*. Novato, CA: New World Library, 1991.

Yoga:
Raskin, D. *Yoga Beats the Blues: Boost Your Mood, Memory, and Concentration with Easy 5, 10, and 20-Minute Yoga Routines*. Gloucester, MA: Fair Winds Press, 2003.

Larson, J. and Howard, K. *Yoga Mom, Buddha Baby: The Yoga Workout for New Moms*. New York: Bantam Books, 2002.

Stanton, L. and Perron, S. *Baby Om: Yoga for Mothers and Babies.* New York: Holt Paperbacks, 2002.

Seasonal Affective Disorder:

Rosenthal, N., MD. *Winter Blues: Everything You Need to Know to Beat Seasonal Affective Disorder.* 4th ed. New York: The Guilford Press, 2012.

Subconscious:

Jensen, C.J. *Beyond the Power of Your Subconscious Mind.* Cardiff, CA: Waterside Publications, 2012.

Postpartum Exercise:

Byrne, H. *Exercise After Pregnancy: How to Look and Feel Your Best.* 2nd ed. Oakland, CA: BeFit-Mom, 2007.

Brin, L. *How to Exercise When You're Expecting: For the 9 Months of Pregnancy and the 5 Months It Takes to Get Your Best Body Back.* New York: Plume, 2011.

Healthy Eating:

Ward, E. *Expect the Best: Your Guide to Healthy Eating Before, During and After Pregnancy.* Hoboken, NJ: John Wiley & Sons, 2009.

Rose, A., Ph.D. and Adams, A., MD. *Rebuild from Depression: A Nutrient Guide Including Depression in Pregnancy and Postpartum.* Hot Springs, CA: Purple Oak Press, 2009.

Journaling:

Adams, K. *Journal to the Self: Twenty-Two Paths to Personal Growth.* New York: Grand Central Publishing, 1990.

Conner, J. *Writing Down Your Soul: How to Activate and Listen to the Extraordinary Voice Within.* San Francisco: Conari Press, 2009.

References

Chapter 1: Sharing Their Stories

"10 Celebrities Who Battled Postpartum Depression." *CBSNews.com.* http://www.cbsnews.com/2300-204_162 -10005857.html

"11 Celebrity Moms Who Battled Postpartum Depression." *The Frisky.* April 14, 2012. http://www.thefrisky.com/2012-04-14 /11-celebrity-moms-who-battled-postpartum -depression/

Ramos, Patricia. "Alanis Morisette Opens Up About Her Postpartum Depression." *Entertainmentwise.* Aug. 28, 2012. http://www.entertainmentwise.com /news/85726/Alanis-Morisette-Opens-Up -About-Her-Postpartum-Depression

Turgeon, Heather. "Gwyneth Paltrow Talks About Her Postpartum Depression." *Stroller Derby* (blog). Jan. 5, 2011. http://blogs.babble.com /strollerderby/2011/01/05/gwyneth-paltrow -talks-about-her-postpartum-depression-take -aways/#more-52670

"Brook Shields: On Her Pregnancy and Postpartum Depression." *iVillage.* May 10, 2005. http://www.ivillage.com/pregnancy-and -postpartum-depression/6-a-127821

Chapter 2: What Is Postpartum Depression?

Dobbs, J., and Titchenal, A. "Postpartum Depression Common, Cause Unknown." *Nutrition ATC.* April 3, 2012. http://www.nutritionatc.hawaii.edu/HO/2012/491.htm

Chapter 3: Overcoming the Stigma of Postpartum Depression — Managing Expectations and Taking Action

Kauppi, C. P., Montgomery, A., Shaikh, and T. White. *Postnatal Depression: When Reality Does Not Match Expectations.* Studbury, Canada: Laurenthian University, 2012.

Nauert, R., PhD. "Postpartum Depression's Effect on the Baby." *PsychCentral.* Reviewed by John M. Grohol, Psy.D. on Aug. 21, 2009. http://psychcentral.com/news/2009/08/21/postpartum-depressions-effect-on-the-baby/7899.html

"Post-Natal Depression." *The Association for Postnatal Illness.* http://apni.org.

"Postpartum Depression: Society, the Individual, and Medicine." University of Ottawa. www.med.uottawa.ca/sim/data/Depression_postpartum_e.htm

Chapter 4: Mind-Body Connection and Postpartum Depression

Center for Natural Alternative Solutions. "Why Do We Not Feel Good." 2006. http://www.natural -alternative-solutions.com

"Depression during and after pregnancy fact sheet." *Womenshealth.gov.* 2009. www.womenshealth.gov/publications/our -publications/fact-sheet/depression-pregnancy .cfm

Healthy Mind Counseling Services, Inc. "Mind/ Body Connection: How your emotions affect your health." 2011. http://healthymindcounseling.blogspot.com

Landers, D. M. "The Influence of Exercise on Mental Health." Arizona State University. Originally published as series 2, no. 12, of the *PCPFS Research Digest.*

Luczaj, S. "Depression and the Mind-Body Connection." *Counsellingresource.com.* 2007. http://counsellingresource.com/features /2007/10/23/depression-mind-body/

Marano, H. E. "When Depression Hurts." *Psychology Today.* July 1, 2002.

"Mind/Body Connection: How Your Emotions Affect Your Health." *FamilyDoctor.org.* 2004; 2010.

Mayo Clinic Staff. "Depression and Anxiety: Exercise Eases Symptoms." *MayoClinic.com.* 2011.

Nutt, D. J. "Relationship of Neurotransmitters to Symptoms of Major Depressive Disorder." *J Clin Psychiatry* 69 Suppl. E1. (2008): 4-7.

"Postpartum Depression and Running: The Mind/Body Connection." *The Complete Running Blog Network.* http://completerunning.com /archives/2008/02/08/postpartum -depression-and-running/

Trivedi, H., MD. "The Link Between Depression and Physical Symptoms: Primary Care Companion." *J Clin Psychiatry* 6 Suppl. 1. (2004): 12-16.

Zeratsky, K., RD, LD. "Junk food blues: Are depression and diet related?" *MayoClinic.com.* 2012.

Chapter 5: Natural Treatment Options for Postpartum Depression

"How Food Benefits Mood." BBC News World Edition. 2002. news.bbc.co.uk/2/hi/health /2264529.stm

"Depression Health Center—Alternative Treatments for Depression." *WebMD.* www.webmd.com /depression/guide/alternative-therapies -depression

Dorman, K. "How Do I Increase Dopamine in the Brain?" *Livestrong.com.* 2011.

"Health Concerns: Depression." *Life Extension.* http://www.lef.org/protocols/emotional _health/depression_01.htm

Mayo Clinic staff. "Postpartum Depression." *MayoClinic.com.* 2010.

Natural Remedies, LLC. "Natural Help 4... Postpartum Depression." 1997-2008.

"Natural Remedies for Postpartum Depression." *Yourpregnancyfriend.com.*

Zeratsky, K., RD, LD. "Junk Food Blues: Are depression and diet related?" *MayoClinic.com.* 2012.

Chapter 6: Informing Your Healthcare Provider

Cox, J. L., J. M. Holden, and R. Sagovsky. "Detection of Postnatal Depression: Development of the 10-item Edinburgh Postnatal Depression Scale." *British Journal of Psychiatry* 150 (1987); 782-86.

Chapter 7: Healthy Diet—You're Still Eating for Two

Edgar, J. "Health Benefits of Green Tea." *WebMD.* 2009.

Ehrlich, S. D., NMD. "Green Tea." *University of Maryland Medical Center.* Last reviewed on Oct. 14, 2011. http://www.umm.edu/altmed /articles/green-tea-000255.htm

Ehrlich, S. D., NMD. "Omega-3 Fatty Acids." *University of Maryland Medical Center.* Last reviewed on May 10, 2011. http://www.umm.edu /altmed/articles/omega-3-000316.htm

"Benefit of Drinking Green Tea." *Harvard Women's Health Watch.* 2002-2012.

Mayo Clinic staff. "Omega-3 Fatty Acids, Fish Oil, Alpha-Linolenic Acid." *MayoClinic.com.* 2011.

Medifast, Inc. "Medifast for Nursing Mothers Meal Plan." 2008.

Park, A. "Why Sleep Deprivation May Lead to Overeating." *Time: Healthland.* 2012.

Peeks, P., MD, MPH, FACP. "Everyday Fitness." *WebMD.* 2010.

Zeratsky, K., RD, LD. "Caffeine: Is it dehydrating or not?" *MayoClinic*.com. 2011.

Chapter 8: Pregnancy, Hormones and Depression

Ahokas, A., MD, Ph.D., J. Kaukoranta, MD, K. Wahlbeck, MD, and M. Aito, MD. "Estrogen Deficiency in Severe Postpartum Depression: Successful Treatment with Sublingual Physiologic 17beta-Estradiol: A Preliminary Study." 2000.

"Acupuncture for Postpartum Depression (Postnatal Depression)." *Acupuncture for Natural Healing.* 1996-2012. www.activeacupuncture.com/postpartum -depression.aspx

Academy of Classical Oriental Sciences. "Treating Post Partum Depression with TCM." *Nelson Daily News.* 2009.

Center for Natural Alternative Solutions. "Bioidentical Hormones." Accessed Jan. 4, 2013. http://www.natural-alternative-solutions.com /site/525077/page/307403

Dach, J, MD. "Bioidentical Hormones for Anxiety and Depression." http://jeffreydach.com /2010/02/19/bioidentical-hormones -relieve-anxiety-by-jeffrey-dach-md.aspx

"Depression during and after pregnancy fact sheet." *Womenshealth.gov.* 2009. www.womenshealth.gov/publications/our -publications/fact-sheet/depression-pregnancy .cfm

Mayo Clinic staff. "Postpartum Depression." *MayoClinic.com.* 2010.

Millehan, J. "Hormones, Mood and Working Out." *Livestrong.com.* 2011.

Palmer, M., E. J. Baugh. "Postpartum Depression." University of Florida IFAS Extension, Department of Family, Youth and Community Sciences. 2008.

"Postpartum Depression and Running: The Mind/Body Connection." *The Complete Running Blog Network.* http://completerunning.com/archives /2008/02/08/postpartum-depression-and -running/

Simpson, J. "Medications Used to Treat Postpartum Depression." *Livestrong.com.* 2010.

WebMD. "Vitex Agnus – Castus." Information provided by Natural Medicines Comprehensive Database Consumer Version. 2009.

"What are Bioidentical Hormones?" *Harvard Women's Health Watch.* 2006.

Chapter 9: Vitamins, Minerals, Herbal Supplements and Food

Ahokas, A., MD, PhD, J. Kaukoranta, MD, Wahlbeck, MD, PhD, and M. Aito. "Estrogen Deficiency in Severe Postpartum Depression: Successful Treatment With Sublingual Physiologic 17beta-Estradiol: A Preliminary Study." *J Clin Psychiatry* 62. (2001):332-36.

Bates, C. Bsc (Hons) Ost. Med. DO, ND. "Post-natal supplement advice for mothers." The Perrymount Osteopathy and Natural Health Clinic.

Center for Natural Alternative Solutions. "Bioidentical Hormones." www.natural-alternative -solutions.com/site/525077/page/3074037

Dach, J, MD. "Bioidentical Hormones for Anxiety and Depression." http://jeffreydach.com /2010/02/19/bioidentical-hormones -relieve-anxiety-by-jeffrey-dach-md.aspx

"Depression and Diet." Depression Health Center. *WebMD.* 2011.

Ehrlich, S. D., NMD. "Herbal Medicine." *University of Maryland Medical Center*. Last reviewed on Oct. 2, 2011. http://www.umm.edu/altmed/articles/herbal-medicine-000351.htm

Ehrlich, S. D., NMD. "Omega-3 fatty acids." *University of Maryland Medical Center*. Last reviewed on May 10, 2011. http://www.umm.edu/altmed/articles/omega-3-000316.htm

Harvard Health Publications. "What are Bioidentical Hormones?" *Harvard Women's Health Watch*. Aug 2006.

La Luz, B. "Preventing Postpartum Hemorrhage Naturally." *Birthfaith.org*. 2010.

Landro, L. "Herbal Supplements Face New Scrutiny." *Wall Street Journal*. Sep. 14, 2012.

Livingston, J. E, MacLeod P. M., and Applegarth D. A. "Vitamin B6 Status in Women with Postpartum Depression." *Am J Clin Nutr* 5. (May 31, 1978):886-91.

Mayo Clinic staff. "Ginkgo (Ginkgo Biloba)." *MayoClinic.com*. 2011.

Mayo Clinic staff. "SAMe." *MayoClinic.com*. Prepared by The Natural Standard Research Collaboration. (Updated 2011.)

Mayo Clinic staff. "Vitamin B6." *MayoClinic.com*. Prepared by The Natural Standard Research Collaboration. (Updated 2011.)

Mayo Clinic staff. "Vitamin B12." *MayoClinic.com.* Prepared by The Natural Standard Research Collaboration. (Updated 2011.)

Medifast, Inc. "Medifast for Nursing Mothers Meal Plan." 2008.

Morgenthaler, T., MD. "Valerian: A Safe and Effective Herbal Sleep Aid?" *MayoClinic.com.* 2012.

"Natural Remedies for Postpartum Depression." *Yourpregnancyfriend.com.*

New Hampshire Breastfeeding Task Force. *A Breastfeeding-Friendly Approach to Depression in New Mothers.* 2009.

Smitt, S. "Calcium Supplements for Breastfeeding Moms." *Livestrong.com.*

"Vitamin D Health Professional Fact Sheet." *Office Of Dietary Supplements–National Institutes of Health* http://ods.od.nih.gov/factsheets /VitaminD-HealthProfessional/

"Vitex Agnus—Castus." *WebMD.* 2012.

Chapter 10: Make Your Move—Exercise and Depression

"Depression During and After Pregnancy Fact Sheet." *Womenshealth.gov.* 2009. www.womenshealth.gov /publications/our-publications/fact-sheet /depression-pregnancy.cfm

Landers, D. M. "The Influence of Exercise on Mental Health." Arizona State University. (Originally published as series 2, no. 12, of the *PCPFS Research Digest.*)

Mayo Clinic staff. "Depression and anxiety: Exercise eases symptoms." *MayoClinic.com.* 2011.

"Postpartum Depression and Running: The Mind/ Body Connection." *The Complete Running Blog Network.* http://completerunning.com /archives/2008/02/08/postpartum -depression-and-running/

Chapter 11: Hypnosis—Using the Power of Your Mind

"Make Easy Changes: Subliminal Learning Works." *Secret Changes.* www.secretchanges.com.

Rude, L., CHt. "Hypnosis." *Secret Changes Hypnosis.* www.secretchangeshypnosis.com

Chapter 12: Take a Break—Relaxation and Stress Management

"Acupuncture: An Alternative and Complementary Medicine Resource Guide." *Alternative Medicine Foundation, Inc.* www.amfoundation.org /acupuncture.htm

Acupuncture World Information Center. "Everything You MUST Know about Acupuncture." www.acupuncture.org/stressanxiety.html

"Alternative Treatments for Depression." *WebMD.* www.webmd.com/depression/guide /alternative-therapies-depression/

Creagan, E. T., MD. "Stress and Weight Gain." *MayoClinic.com.* 2011.

"Dopamine." *Psychology Today.* www.psychologytoday.com/basics/dopamine

Hall-Flavin, D., MD. "Stress and Hair Loss: Are They Related?" *MayoClinic.com.* 2010.

Kuchinskas, S. "Meditation Heals Body and Mind." *WebMD.* 2005-2007.

Leonard, C. "How Does Massage Therapy Relieve Stress?" *Livestrong.com.* 2010.

"Major Research Areas." *Integrative Medicine at Yale.* http://cam.yale.edu/research/areas.aspx

Mayo Clinic staff. "Hypnosis." *MayoClinic.com.* 2009.

Mayo Clinic staff. "Meditation: A Simple, Fast Way to Reduce Stress." *MayoClinic.com.* 2011.

Mayo Clinic staff. "Stress Symptoms: Effects on Your Body, Feelings and Behavior." *MayoClinic.com.* 2011.

Wong, C. "Acupuncture for Depression." *About. com.* 2012. http://altmedicine.about.com/od/depression/a/acupuncture_depression.htm

"After Pregnancy Weight Loss: Yoga After Pregnancy." *Yoga From A To Z.* www.yoga-from-a-to-z.com/after-pregnancy-weight.html

Scott, E., MS. "Cortisol and Stress: How to Stay Healthy." *About.com Guide.* 2011.

Yexley, M. J. "Treating Postpartum Depression with Hypnosis: Addressing Specific Symptoms Presented by the Client." *American Journal of Clinical Hypnosis* 3. (2007).

Chapter 13: Breathe—Herbs and Aromatherapy

Allardice, P. *The Art Of Aromatherapy.* Avanel, New Jersey: Crescent Books, 2002.

Ehrlich, S. D., NMD. "Aromatherapy." *University of Maryland Medical Center.* Last reviewed on Aug. 9, 2011. http://www.umm.edu/altmed /articles/aromatherapy-000347.htm

Nordqvist, C. "What is Aromatherapy? The Theory Behind Aromatherapy." *Medical News Today.* (2009).

"Why Aromatherapy Works." Paper presented in Massage Continuing Education for the Apollo Correspondence Courses. 2007.

Chapter 14: Speak Up—The Power of Therapy

"14 Tips to Prevent Postpartum Depression." *AskMoxie.org.* 2007.

Mayo Clinic staff. "Postpartum Depression." *MayoClinic.com.* 2010.

Mayo Clinic staff. "Psychotherapy." *MayoClinic.com.*

Natural Remedies, LLC. "Natural Help 4... Postpartum Depression." 1997-2008.

"Post-Natal Depression." *The Association for Postnatal Illness.* apni.org

Chapter 15: Brighten Up Your Life—Light Therapy

Mayo Clinic staff. "Light Therapy." *MayoClinic.com.* 2010.

Chapter 16: Take Notes—The Art of Journaling

Desy, P. "Readers Respond: Tips for Writing and Journal Keeping as a Form of Therapy." *About. com.* healing.about.com/u/ua/journalkeeping /journal-tips.htm

Rainer, T. and Nin, A. *The New Diary.* New York: Penguin Group, 2004.

Chapter 17: Rest Up—A Guide for Sleep

"14 Tips to Prevent Postpartum Depression." *AskMoxie.org.* 2007.

Jaret, P. "New Research Shows that Treating Insomnia Can Help Treat Depression." *WebMD.* Reviewed by Brunilda Nazario, MD. 2012.

Landers, D.M. "The Influence of Exercise on Mental Health." Arizona State University. Originally published as series 2, no. 12 of the *PCPFS Research Digest.*

Mindell, A. *Sleeping Through the Night, Revised Edition: How Infants, Toddlers, and Their Parents Can Get a Good Night's Sleep.* New York: HarperCollins, 2005.

Natural Remedies, LLC. "Natural Help 4... Postpartum Depression." 1997-2008.

Park, A. "Why Sleep Deprivation May Lead to Overeating." *Time: Healthland.* 2012.

Peeks, P. "Everyday Fitness." *WebMD.* 2010.

"Post-Natal Depression." *The Association for Postnatal Illness.* apni.org.

Rude, L., CHt. "Aromatherapy for Sleep." *Postpartum Living.* www.postpartum-living.com.

About the Author

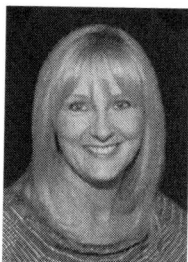

LAURA RUDE is an author, Washington State certified hypnotherapist and founder of the website Postpartum-Living.com, a resource for new mothers and their families who find themselves dealing with postpartum depression. Because of the immense number of women who struggle with the disorder and the devastating effect it has on new mothers and their families, Laura began researching the topic and bringing together information and creating a place to share stories and resources. Laura has worked with a vast number of clients in her hypnotherapy practice and witnessed how a natural and utterly side-effect-free therapy like hypnosis can benefit those suffering with various afflictions of both body and mind. Laura is an avid student of the subconscious mind and has researched natural methods for dealing with depression, stress and anxiety. She discovered that many new moms preferred a natural, drug-free approach to treating their postpartum depression but found little available to them. Through her extensive research, she has written this book and created an easy-to-follow six-week program, implementing natural and holistic methods for combating this disorder.

Laura is married with one son and lives near Seattle, Washington.

Help Yourself!

As an owner of this book, you can receive free products to support your postpartum wellness! Just log onto: www.Postpartum-Living.com/program, click on the "free products for book owners" link and input the code words, "new mother blueprint".

Help a Friend!

If you know someone who could benefit from owning a copy of this book, please direct her to: www.Postpartum-Living.com/book.

Index

W

Made in the USA
Lexington, KY
06 January 2014